The Safe and Sure Way to Reduce

The Safe and Sure Way to Reduce

BY **GAYNOR MADDOX**

RANDOM HOUSE

NEW YORK

FOR Dorothy and Patrick

FOREWORD

REPORTERS are educators, and the public is their audience. In another realm, good scientists are often good educators, but seldom are they good reporters—except to a select audience.

All too often the reporter has no opportunity—or adequate time and patience—to gather information that is both interesting and accurate from the best scientific sources, and then systematically to interpret research progress to the public. Reporting science to the public, nevertheless, has become an important new profession.

Gaynor Maddox merits a "Thank You" and congratulations from nutrition scientists and from the public, alike, for his persistence, skill and sincerity in searching for the most authoritative sources of information about foods and nutrition. Equal credit is merited for the success achieved in his press columns and in the preparation of this book, as a guide for the public. His interpretation of ideas and practices relative to the use of foods, in a manner that holds the respect of leading scientists and wins acceptance by the public, is an important achievement.

CHARLES GLEN KING,

Executive Director—Nutrition Foundation
Professor of Chemistry—Columbia University

ACKNOWLEDGMENTS

TWO MEN, both physically trim, Boyd Lewis, executive editor and vice-president of the Newspaper Enterprise Association, and Dr. Charles Glen King, executive director of the Nutrition Foundation and professor of chemistry, Columbia University, supplied me with the initial self-confidence needed to write this book.

Three years ago Mr. Lewis, noted for his readiness to break editorial precedent at the drop of a better idea, encouraged me to write my first series on weight control based exclusively on the latest researches of outstanding scientists in the field of obesity, rather than on the untested theories of popular self-styled experts. The marked success of this and subsequent series proved, as he had foreseen, that a large segment of the overweight public was fed up on pseudo-science and wanted the facts.

Dr. King, pre-eminent in the field of nutritional research, recognized in these NEA articles a means to carry the findings of research laboratories into American homes. He urged me to develop them into a book. He not only opened reluctant laboratory doors to my inquiry but during the year and a half it took to write this book acted as my uncompromising mentor and was always there to bolster my self-confidence when the enormity of the assignment seemed overpowering.

To both these men, each distinguished in his special field, I am deeply and understandably indebted.

I owe much, also, to Dr. Fredrick J. Stare, chairman, Department of Nutrition, Harvard University, who has spent long hours clarifying many of the ideas expressed in these pages. Dr. Martha F. Trulson and Dr. Jean Mayer, of the same department at Harvard, gave factual help in my efforts to understand why people get fat and what can be done about it. So did Dr. W. H. Sebrell, Jr., director of the Institute of Nutrition Sciences at Columbia University; Dr. Alfred E. Fischer, Department of Pediatrics, Mount Sinai Hospital; Dr. Herbert Pollack, American Heart Association; Dr. Norman Jolliffe, New York City Department of Health; Dr. Ruth Leverton, Department of Human Nutrition, United States Department of Agriculture; Mrs. Dorothea E. Turner, University of Chicago; and Dr. Conrad A. Elvehjem, formerly professor of biochemistry and now president of the University of Wisconsin.

Many thanks are due also to David Quinlan and Paul Lapolla for their insistent loyalty, and to Mrs. Thelma Pollen of the American Dietetic Association for her untiring help in supplying scientific papers and introducing me to many member dietitians who have contributed to my understanding of the subject. To Mrs. Elizabeth K. Caso, Harvard School of Public Health and chairman, 1959, of the Diet Therapy Section of the American Dietetic Association, not only I but also my readers are indebted for her thorough technical checking of the manuscript.

Without the patient daily editorial assistance and expert criticism of my wife Dorothy, and her co-operation in testing in our own home the diets and principles advocated in these pages, the job could not have been done. Thanks, too, to my young son Patrick, who, after reading the manuscript, stated that he was convinced and had determined then and there never to let himself get fat.

CONTENTS

PART III

Successful Reducing Diets Use Familiar Foods

PART IV

Sound Nutrition Blocks Overweight

PART V

Misinformation and Superstition Can Thwart the Dieter

The Safe and Sure Way to Reduce

INTRODUCTION

Lose Pounds
but Keep
Your Head

THIS IS an optimistic book. It is based on the sure foundation that common sense, a normal amount of will power, a desire to enjoy living, and current researches in biochemistry and nutrition promise you a brighter prospect for a long and useful life and a more slender body.

Although traffic jams and taxes are still the lot of man, obesity does not have to be. Admittedly, our gross national overweight would seem to deny it. Slenderness based on health, however, can be like liberty—the reward of unending vigilance and a large measure of "do something about it."

Strip your clothes off. Stand in front of a full-length mirror. Take a long, hard, uncompromising look at your body.

That private moment may be the beginning of wisdom for you.

You are overweight? One out of every five Americans over thirty years of age is overweight. You bulge? You may be obese—that means more than 10 pounds above your desirable weight for your height. You are shocked at the rolls of evidence that have slowly crept up on you.

Today, we are living in an age when diabetes, cardiovascular and other diseases associated with overweight exact a heavy toll. Therefore, any excess poundage reflected in that mirror may be a health hazard. Nor is it alluring, either. So whether your basic urge is to lengthen your life span or improve your appearance, you are looking at what you must banish.

Undoubtedly you have been eating too much for a long time,

maybe all your life. So have far too many of us. We are all spoiled
with coddling in a land of plenty—our record of 20 percent
incidence of gross malnutrition in the form of overweight alone
should jar us from any complacency.

The chances are you don't get enough physical exercise. Few
of us do. In other words, most of us follow the cultural pattern of
our times. We get fat not because we are different. We get fat
because we are *not* different.

Yet that does not release you from the consequences of overweight. In self-defense you must do something to correct it. However, it is important not to burden yourself with an undue sense
of guilt.

Reduce within Your Cultural Pattern

Despite the fact that our cultural pattern is supercharged with
calories, it's the only pattern in which we can live and carry on
a normal life. A diet pattern that derails us socially can become
an emotional risk. Also it is destined to be short-lived.

But you can maintain a desirable weight without trying to
escape from the world you live in. Because obesity has become
such a large-scale health problem many of our outstanding
scientists are dedicating their lives to the discovery of its causes,
cost, prevention and cure. There is a growing mass of reliable
material, based on research in clinics, hospitals and university
laboratories, on the physiological, nutritional and psychiatric
aspects of overweight.

To lose unwanted pounds and still live in the world of men,
plan your reducing schedule on the findings of these accredited
researchers. Use this book as the liaison between their laboratory
and clinical findings and your bathroom scales.

The research done proves the importance of intelligent planning of meals, rather than starvation or crash diets, as the best
path back to normal weight and health. Researchers define the
science of nutrition as the science of food in its relation to life
and health, and point out that loss of weight alone is not the full
measure of a successful long-term diet. If you can lose weight

and at the same time remain emotionally stable and at physical peak, only then are the odds in your favor.

That means your diet is made up of a variety of foods which in proper relation to each other, and adapted both to your way of living and your budget, supply the nutrients needed for optimum health. Of course, two other elements are essential for success—a realistic understanding of your need to get down to and stay at your desirable weight, plus a self-induced and reasonable amount of determination to do it.

Let's face it. Good advice is the hardest thing for people to take. So we'll make ours as brief as practicable. Eat a variety of foods, go easy on fats, pass up seconds, avoid binges on any particular food, and don't get the idea that a pound of steak and three martinis constitute a reducing diet.

And, like growing up normally, growing down to your desirable weight takes a long time.

Food the Basis of Effective Diets

Food, not starvation, is the basis for weight reduction with built-in permanence. By food is meant just what you have always thought it meant—items on your grocer's shelves. *It does not mean so-called health or natural foods, pills, vitamin supplements or drugs.* These are expensive, may be dangerous unless recommended by a physician experienced in weight control, and do not help re-educate your appetite. Save the money you might be tempted to spend on these overpriced gimmicks and buy yourself a pair of walking shoes.

Steak, potatoes, bread, cake and pie—these foods are woven into our pattern of living. In many parts of the country the same is true of cocktails, highballs, beer and wine. All these and others can be included in any reducing menus.

Your diet, to be effective, must be made up of foods you enjoy, foods you can easily find on your grocer's shelves and foods you can afford. But how often you use them, and in what amounts, is a horse of a different color. *Modern nutrition, scientific weight control and emotional stability are the three regulating factors.*

Go Easy on Fats

Because fats are the most concentrated source of calories, they are easiest to restrict. However, moderate use of them is important for health and food enjoyment.

An excess of saturated (hard) fats may be proved to predispose you to hardening of the arteries. But this question is still far from being settled. In any event, according to present evidence, the saturated fats can readily be balanced in the diet by unsaturated or salad oil types of fat—not any kind, but the correct kind.

In any case, it is just common sense, of course, to be moderate in the amount of fat in your diet. Many of us have been in the habit of getting 40 to 45 percent of our calories from fat. You can have good meals—yes, even gourmet meals—and still stick to a 30 percent maximum.

There is no such thing as a "fattening" food. It's the total number of calories in *all* the food you eat that counts. No single food is essential in these weight-control programs, nor is any single food forbidden. Eating too much is the problem. What calories you don't burn up, pile up.

Your unsympathetic mirror will confirm this. Those extra inches around your middle were a long time coming. Calories are sneaky, like wolves wrapped in mouth-watering clothing.

Excess Pounds Sneak Up on You

Emphasizing the sneaky character of excess calories that finally snap the buttons, Dr. Fredrick J. Stare, M.D., Ph.D., Harvard University Department of Nutrition, warns that a healthy man or woman does not become overweight between Christmas and New Year's but between New Year's and Christmas.

Dr. Charles Glen King, executive director, Nutrition Foundation, also stresses that putting on or taking off pounds is no matter of gastronomic sleight of hand. "The longer you have been overweight," he says, "the harder it will be to get back to what you should weigh."

After the age of twenty-five, a healthy man or woman needs

about 5 percent less food every ten years to keep his body functioning at peak. But, unhappily, most of us go right on eating the same amount, often more.

Older people, necessarily less active, need still fewer calories. If grandparents hope to remain healthy and attractive, they should eat much less than their grandchildren, particularly if they hope to live long enough to enjoy their great-grandchildren.

The moment of final decision to do something about your figure (and your basic health) can be a deeply upsetting one for you. Frustration, guilt complexes, and even desperation may scuttle your normal way of thinking. But these are poor ingredients for a successful program.

Admittedly, and this fact should be faced head-on, the battle against obesity is a tough one. Dr. James Hundley, of the National Institutes of Health, warns, "Often a surprisingly high percentage succeed in losing weight. But only a few maintain it."

Drastic Reducing of Food Dangerous

Dr. King adds, "The solution to overweight, now one of our major national health problems, is the readjustment of our way of eating to modern life and what we have learned about food values."

Drastic reductions in food, unless medically advised, or bizarre emphasis on one particular type of food as against another, may upset the nutritional and emotional balance of the dieter and put a substitute burden on the heart. So what does it profit you to lose a few pounds if you lose your health and sense of wellbeing? Or for a man to be able to tighten his belt, if, at the same time, with his free hand he reaches out for drugs, alcohol, or more cigarettes?

PART I

CALORIES
AND
WEIGHT
CONTROL

CHAPTER 1

Unused Calories
Turn to Fat

MOST OF US are overweight simply because we eat too much. We take on more fuel for living than our bodies require. That extra food bites the hand it feeds. What fuel our bodies don't burn up in daily activity turns to fat. It's as devastatingly simple as that.

For example—roughly, the average man who leads a sedentary life requires around 2,400 calories a day. Therefore, if he eats 2,900 calories, he is taking aboard 500 more calories than he can use. Those 500 extra calories clutter the deck. At this rate, in a week he has overloaded himself with 3,500 calories.

Those unused 3,500 calories a week are like the man who came to dinner. They stick around. Actually, 3,500 calories are the equivalent of 1 pound of body fat. So if he continues to over-eat by only 500 calories a day, he will be 52 pounds above his desirable weight in a year.

For a woman with a washing machine, push-button kitchen or sedentary job, about 2,000 calories a day are required to maintain figure and fitness. If she eats 500 calories more than the basic 2,000 needed, she too will gain a pound a week, over 4 pounds a month, and 52 pounds a year.

Dress Sizes Change with Pounds

Let's translate those excess pounds resulting from eating more food than the body needs into manufacturers' dress sizes. According to experts of the United States Department of Commerce, there is a 10-pound difference between small sizes, a 12- to 14-pound difference between medium sizes, and a difference of 16 or more pounds between large sizes. Therefore, an increase of 52 pounds a year (eating only 500 calories more a day than your body needs) will mean for a woman, no matter what her build, a considerable outlay every year for new dresses in which she can breathe more comfortably.

Now, as surely as the fact that what goes up must come down, if you cut 500 calories out of your daily food intake, you can *lose* a pound a week, over 4 pounds a month, or 52 pounds a year, no matter what you weigh at this moment.

Of course, if you cut 1,000 calories out of your daily food intake, you will lose 2 pounds a week; if 1,500 calories, 3 pounds a week. You can cut down as much as you desire provided you have no objections to losing your health and your life along with pounds.

A word of warning—a little cold water to dash on your frantic desire to slim down in a few days—most physicians and nutritionists in obesity clinics advise against cutting out more than 1,000 calories a day, except in extreme cases.

Think of Calories in Terms of Familiar Foods

What does 500 calories look like in terms of things you enjoy eating? Here are a few familiar examples: one wedge of apple pie à la mode; two waffles with two pats of butter and syrup; two large doughnuts, a sweet roll and a pat of butter. All these items are perfectly good foods despite high-calorie content. On the other hand, a satisfying and nutritionally balanced dinner of fillet of sole baked in milk, a parsley potato, cooked carrots, lettuce, tangerine and cottage cheese salad, fresh fruit gelatin and coffee or tea adds up to only 550 calories. So does this man-sized breakfast: grapefruit, coffee cake with nuts and icing, a scrambled egg, coffee or tea with sugar.

All the above discussion of why you get fat and what calories look like in dinner-table terms is admittedly oversimplified. Nevertheless, so far as it goes, it is based on the most recent scientific findings. Therefore, take it as gospel that you are overweight because you eat too much.

Overeating the Major Cause of Obesity

But it will follow as the night the day, many of you will say, "Oh, I am different."

"My glands"; "Inherited tendency to fat"; "I don't eat very much but my body turns everything into fat"—these are standard self-deceptions.

Once you have accepted the fact that overeating is the major cause of obesity, your feet are on the path to effective long-term weight control. But you have taken only the first step.

CHAPTER 2

Calories Necessary
in All Diets

THE SIMPLE reason for having more pounds than you want is that you eat more calories than your body needs. But that does not mean calories is a dreaded word.

To live, you must have food, and food means calories. But not necessarily more than you need. So if you are too fat and want to lose some of it, reorganize your eating habits. Cut down on calories but do not cut them out.

Not starvation, not martyrdom, but a sound reorganization of your daily eating is the only common-sense way to lose weight, keep your health and get fun out of life—three vital objectives to most people.

That formula is the foundation of modern scientific weight control. So plan your diet accordingly if you want lasting results.

Jet, miracle and wonder diets have the appeal of old-fashioned melodrama. They are equally corny. Avoid them.

Weight Control and Nutrition Inseparable

Like love and marriage, effective weight control and nutrition go together. Nutrition is what you find in your supermarket. No voodoo items required. Magic and self-deception don't belong.

To lose weight without losing your head, you need three things: (1) a reasonable amount of will power, (2) a workable knowledge of nutrition, (3) a sturdy market cart.

Unfortunately, nutrition, like virtue, does not seem exciting. But whereas virtue is its own reward, the rewards of nutrition are better growth and health, more zest for living, and physical independence. None of these necessarily interferes with a life of virtue.

The science of nutrition is the science of food and its relation to life and health. The ABC's of nutrition are to eat a wide variety of good foods every day.

If reorganizing your eating habits in order to lose weight and keep your health while doing it is of prime importance to you, then take time to learn what follows. It is the road map to permanent weight control.

There are six main food groups which make up a balanced diet: carbohydrates, fats, proteins, vitamins, minerals and water. Practically every familiar food you eat contains several or all of these groups in varying amount.

It makes no difference whether you are on a 2,000- or 1,000-calorie diet; the rule holds. *All* these nutrients are needed for nutritional balance.

Eat from Four Food Groups Every Day

Now let's translate that scientific formula into market-list terms. You must eat some food every day from *each* of these groupings of familiar foods:

1. Meat, poultry, fish, cheese, milk.
2. Vegetables and fruits (including some citrus such as oranges and grapefruit—or tomato juice) and some dark green leafy or yellow vegetable.
3. Cereals, potatoes, macaroni or rice, bread.
4. Fats—butter or margarine, edible oils.

Does all this talk about eating things like meat and potatoes and vegetables puzzle you when you want to lose weight? Don't let it. Although the purpose of this book is to help you lose un-needed fat, it does not aim to destroy your appeal. A skinny, nervous, petulant woman (in this case, meaning an under-nourished one) is not attractive. Nor is a lean but frustrated man (the fellow who is afraid to eat because he may lose his boyish figure). Lasting weight control is health control. To a large degree, health control is impossible without sound nutrition; sound nutrition is impossible without good food; and good food is impossible without calories.

Enjoy Favorite Foods in Your Diet

Of course good nutrition and effective weight control require limitation of calories to the amount needed by your body to function best. Limitation of calories, however, does not mean you have to eat foods you dislike. It means further (but within moderation) that you can include some of almost every food you like in your weight-control diet and still stay within your calorie limitations.

Now that you realize calories are respectable, let's get better acquainted with them.

CHAPTER 3

Calories Are
a Personal Matter

THE SCIENTIFIC definition of a calorie is this: enough heat to raise the temperature of a pint of water by four degrees. In terms of your own body, a calorie is a measure of fuel that helps keep you going. But if you take on more fuel than the engine burns up, then you get into trouble. The trouble is fat. Yes, just that —fat. Every calorie over the amount needed by your particular body is stored on your frame, too often around the hips or on your belly.

Another way of saying all this is that calories are what you must eat enough of to stay active and well; what you must not eat too much of unless you like being outsize; and what if you don't eat enough of you'll lose your health and vitality and look scrawny.

How many calories do you need? That is a decidedly personal question. If you are tall and large-boned, you'll need more than a petite neighbor with a very delicate frame. If you chop wood for a living or drive a truck, you'll need much more than a bank clerk. If you are sixty-five years old, you need many fewer than your twenty-year-old grandson. And you'll probably need many fewer than your grandmother did at the same age, because she didn't run her home in the era of labor-saving devices.

Number Needed Determined by Body Structure and Age

In other words, activity, occupation, body structure and age are factors in determining how many calories a day you need.

For all practical purposes, if you understand calories in terms of customary foods, you can handle your own weight-control

17

problems. For example, an average slice of bread contains about 65 calories and an average pat of butter, 45. So you know that a slice of buttered bread totals 110 calories. A cup of coffee or tea adds no calories to your meal, but for each teaspoon of sugar you stir into it, the total of calories will jump by 16 calories. Four ounces of orange juice contain 55 calories but the same amount of tomato juice has only 25.

However, don't turn to a table and try to learn and memorize the number of calories in all the different foods you eat during the day. That is laborious and most likely will be frustrating. Modern experts in diet do not advise it. Furthermore, it is not necessary.

Avoid Frustrating Calorie Tables

The more practical and approved method of calorie bookkeeping is based on planning meals with exchange lists. All the foods you will need are divided into six basic nutritional groups called exchange groups. Each food within a single list contains about the same number of calories as any other food in the list.

This method, developed by the American Dietetic Association and the American Diabetes Association, takes the mathematical strain out of meal planning for a long-term weight-control program. It also encourages the use of a wide variety of foods daily, thereby avoiding the monotony which can easily discourage the dieter. For the complete guide to this method of calorie bookkeeping in kitchen terms, see Part VI.

You need also a working knowledge of the number of calories you yourself need to be well fed and well shaped. Let's call it a rule of thumb, because the figures used are approximate, based on overall averages.

The table following gives the daily calorie needs for moderately active men and women twenty-five years old. The year twenty-five is the base, because from that age on you will need fewer calories, roughly about 5 percent fewer calories for each ten more years of age. For example, if you are a woman and at twenty-five needed 2,600 calories, at age forty you will need 7½ percent less, or 2,505 a day, to maintain your normal weight.

The Older You Are, the Fewer Calories You Need

Before studying these tables, be warned that many experts in obesity consider their allowances a trifle overgenerous. So if you must make a miscalculation, make it on the minus side.

And bear in mind also that these tables are based on the calorie needs of moderately active twenty-five-year-old men and

Calorie Needs for Moderately Active Twenty-five-Year-Old Men and Women*

YOUR WEIGHT IN POUNDS	APPROXIMATE NUMBER OF CALORIES NEEDED DAILY	
	Men	Women
100		2,000
105		2,100
110		2,100
115	2,700	2,200
120	2,800	2,300
125	2,900	2,400
130	3,000	2,400
135	3,100	2,500
140	3,100	2,600
145	3,200	2,600
150	3,300	2,700
155	3,400	2,800
160	3,500	2,800
165	3,500	2,900
170	3,600	2,900
175	3,700	
180	3,800	
185	3,900	
190	3,900	
195	4,000	
200	4,100	

* Based on information in Recommended Dietary Allowances. National Research Council, Washington, D. C.

women. The longer you live, the less you need to eat if you hope
to live still longer.

Incidentally, a moderately active person could be a home-
maker, a sales person, a factory worker. Persons who are more
active will need more calories; those who live a more "sit-down"
life, such as the office worker, will need fewer.

So much, temporarily, for the number of calories you need to
maintain your weight; that is, to prevent yourself from getting
any heavier than you are at the moment.

Learn Nutritional Value of Calories

Now let us examine the nutritional value of calories. Don't be
tricked into thinking that knowing how many calories there are
in a serving of food is enough. Calories, like people, are known
by the company they keep. Company, in this regard, means
nutritional values. All foods contain calories, but some do not
contain essential protein, fat, carbohydrates, minerals and
vitamins. Sugar, for example, contains only calories (energy),
and no other nutritional elements. Such calories are called
"empty calories." Alcohol, sugar, cooking fats and some candies
are in that category.

Some "empty calories" have a place in a scientific weight-
reduction program, if only for the pleasure value, but only in
moderate amounts. On the other hand, although protective foods
such as meat, dairy products, cereals, fruit and vegetables and
fats contain calories in varying degree—in fact, some in large
degree—they must be included in even highly restricted diets
because of their nutritional importance. Cutting these basic
foods out of your weight-control menus, thereby depriving
yourself of the elements needed for health, happiness and the
will to live, just because they contain calories, is very much
like cutting off your nose to spite your face—even if it's a very
plump face.

Therefore, in planning your special menus, go easy on the
"empty calories." You don't have to cut them out entirely, because lack of them might make you feel dissatisfied and discourage you from sticking to your diet. But take it easy.

A Basic and Flexible 1,500-Calorie Diet Pattern

The table below gives you a graphic picture of the importance of protective foods in a 1,500-calorie diet despite their calories. Even though this carefully planned, nutritionally balanced menu pattern contains most of the foods you enjoy, including sugar and butter, it will help you lose weight without depriving you of any nutritional elements. It is a far cry from many fad diets that endanger your health and cost you a lot of money.

Basic 1,500-Calorie Diet Pattern

FOR THE DAY	AMOUNT	CALORIES
Milk, non-fat	1 pint	170
Meat, Fish, Fowl, Eggs, Hard Cheese	8 ounces	576
Breads, Cereals, Noodles, Potatoes, etc.	6 servings	390
Vegetables	3 or 4 servings	40
Fruits (no sugar added)	4 servings	160
Sugar	2 teaspoons	32
Fats (butter, margarine, oils and shortenings)	2 teaspoons	90
APPROXIMATE TOTAL CALORIES		1,458

Remember, this basic outline is flexible and allows for variation. The quantity of calories contained is a rough estimate. The protein category includes beef, chicken, fish (seafood), veal, lamb and other cuts of meat. One egg is equal to an ounce of meat, and for the purposes of this outline, an ounce of hard cheese can also be used as the equivalent of an ounce of meat.

Using this menu pattern, experiment with menus that you, personally, enjoy. To anyone who needs to lose weight and keep it lost, the first rule is to learn what to eat rather than what not to eat.

CHAPTER 4

Estimate Pounds
You Should Lose

YOUR MIRROR and your bathroom scales can tell you dramatically how much overweight you are—maybe not to the exact number of pounds, but certainly near enough for all practical purposes of reducing. In fact, this whole business of reducing is a common-sense matter. To be effective and long-lasting, all your weight-control efforts must be free of panic, self-torture, neurosis and compulsions.

Actually, getting down to your desirable weight and staying there is much more a way of life (maybe a new way of life) than it is a flagellation of your bulging body.

So don't feel too embarrassed by that thickness back of your neck, by that much too prominent abdomen, by the unbecoming padding on your hips. About fifty million other American men and women are overweight, too. In fact, overweight has become our No. 1 health problem. Therefore, instead of feeling guilty and ashamed because of your fatness, realize that it raises a problem for you shared by millions of others. It is unfortunate, not criminal.

Use Pinch Test for Obesity

Now, to convince yourself that something must be done, pinch yourself into dynamic resolve that action is needed—for health, for looks, for more zest.

Pinch yourself on the back of the upper arm, or below the shoulder blade. You don't have to be a scientist to feel the difference between fat and muscle. If the fold pinched up between your thumb and forefinger is about an inch thick, then don't argue. You are overweight.

About that spare tire on the stomach. Lie flat on your back and relax. Does it disappear? If not, then you are overweight.

This "rule of thumb" test will give you an honest practical answer to "Am I really fat?" If you are still in doubt about it, however, move over to your bathroom scale.

Weigh yourself accurately without clothes. Next, accurately measure your height, without shoes.

When you know your weight in pounds, and your height in feet and inches, you can estimate what your desirable weight should be.

Estimate only, remember. To figure your ideal weight would require calculation and weighing beyond the skill of the layman. So settle for a rough estimate of your desirable weight.

For women: depending on whether you have a slight, medium or large frame, allow from 100 to 110 pounds for the first 5 feet of height. Add to that total 5 pounds more for each extra inch.

If you are under five feet, subtract 5 pounds for every inch under five feet.

Base Estimate on Body Weight

Let's take an example. A woman is 5 feet 2 inches tall. She wears small sizes in gloves and shoes, indicating that she has a slight frame. To figure her desirable weight, allow 100 pounds for the first five feet, then add 10 pounds for the 2 inches over 5 feet. The answer is 110 pounds.

If another woman, the same height, has large bone structure, broad shoulders, large hands and feet, allow 110 pounds for the first 5 feet, then 5 pounds more for each inch over 5 feet. Her desirable weight is 120 pounds.

For a man: allow 110 pounds for the first 5 feet of height, and 5½ pounds for each inch over 5 feet. For example, for a man 5 feet 8 inches tall, allow 110 pounds for the first 5 feet and 5½ pounds for each of the additional 8 inches. His estimated desirable weight is then 154 pounds.

Desirable Weights for Men and Women of Ages Twenty-five and Over*

MEN

HEIGHT (WITH 1-INCH HEELS)	WEIGHT IN POUNDS AS ORDINARILY DRESSED		
	Small frame	Medium frame	Large frame
5 ft. 2 in.	116-125	124-133	131-142
5 ft. 3 in.	119-128	127-136	133-144
5 ft. 4 in.	122-132	130-140	137-149
5 ft. 5 in.	126-136	134-144	141-153
5 ft. 6 in.	129-139	137-147	145-157
5 ft. 7 in.	133-143	141-151	149-162
5 ft. 8 in.	136-147	145-156	153-166
5 ft. 9 in.	140-151	149-160	157-170
5 ft. 10 in.	144-155	153-164	161-175
5 ft. 11 in.	148-159	157-168	165-180
6 ft. 0 in.	152-164	161-173	169-185
6 ft. 1 in.	157-169	166-178	174-190
6 ft. 2 in.	163-175	171-184	179-196
6 ft. 3 in.	168-180	176-189	184-202

WOMEN

HEIGHT (WITH 1-INCH HEELS)	WEIGHT IN POUNDS AS ORDINARILY DRESSED		
	Small frame	Medium frame	Large frame
4 ft. 11 in.	104-111	110-118	117-127
5 ft. 0 in.	105-113	112-120	119-129
5 ft. 1 in.	107-115	114-122	121-131
5 ft. 2 in.	110-118	117-125	124-135
5 ft. 3 in.	113-121	120-128	127-138
5 ft. 4 in.	116-125	124-132	131-142
5 ft. 5 in.	119-128	127-135	133-145
5 ft. 6 in.	123-132	130-140	138-150
5 ft. 7 in.	126-136	134-144	142-154
5 ft. 8 in.	129-139	137-147	145-158
5 ft. 9 in.	133-143	141-151	149-162
5 ft. 10 in.	136-147	145-155	152-166
5 ft. 11 in.	139-150	148-158	155-169

* Tables from Metropolitan Life Insurance Co.

Just a note of warning. Large frame means large bone structure and muscle development. It does not mean heaviness or spread caused by fat. A football player may be massive and not have an extra ounce of fat on his frame. On the other hand, a fat man can be just as massive but still have only a moderate build. The difference between him and the football player is that he is padded on the inside while the player is padded only on the outside, if he is still doing active work.

There is another way to estimate your desirable weight according to your height and build. Study the table opposite.

The weights given in this table are a little on the generous side. The calculations were made on men and women fully dressed. But the calculations were made several years ago when men and women wore much heavier clothing than they do today.

Another fact to remember is that this table gives *average* desirable weights. As you may not fit into the average, the figures given for your height and build may only approximate your desirable weight. Even so, they will be near enough for all practical purposes.

Once you have established your desirable weight, then subtract it from your present weight. The answer will be the number of pounds you have to shed.

In terms of health, those extra pounds are a burden and a threat. Actuarial tables of life insurance companies indicate that people who are 20 percent overweight die at a rate 17 percent higher than those of normal weight, and those 30 percent overweight, at a rate 34 percent higher. If vanity is not enough to get you started on your weight-control program, then ponder those insurance figures. While you are doing it, hang a bag on a rope around your neck and fill it with enough pebbles to equal the number of pounds you must lose. A little gruesome, maybe, but so is the thought of dying before your time because you eat too much.

CHAPTER 5

Lose Weight Slowly
but Steadily

YOU NOW know about how many pounds you should lose. But
before you embark on a weight-control program, have a heart-
to-heart talk with yourself. Are you convinced of the soundness
of a long-term undertaking for better looks and better health
instead of repeated crash diets? Are you eager to re-educate
yourself in better eating habits? Are you emotionally secure
enough to undertake this program and to follow it enthusias-
tically? Will your family co-operate with you? Have you checked
with your doctor as to whether you should reduce or not and
how much?

Remember, this is not to be a shotgun wedding. Fear, fashion
and fads are not enough to spark a continuing program. This
is for keeps. It is for permanent weight control for the rest of
your life, for a happier, more vital and longer life.

If your answers have been "yes," then take that bag of excess
pounds with one hand and a strong grip on your will power
with the other, and get going.

How fast should you lose those excess pounds? Do you want
an honest answer? Then take the advice of all researchers in
obesity. Be a tortoise, not a hare.

Limit Weight Loss from 1 to 3 Pounds a Week

For a lasting program, limit your weekly loss to from 1 to 3
pounds, researchers advise, knowing from years of clinical experience that the faster you lose weight, the quicker you are
liable to regain it.

The reason why slow weight loss is recommended by

physicians and dietitians with experience in obesity is that the dieter then will be less likely to go off his diet and put on weight again. The history of crash and fad dieters is that they lose with drastic speed but almost invariably, after a short period of self-imposed starvation, regain their excess weight.

These on-again, off-again dieters, who gain, lose, gain, may induce high blood pressure by repeated gainings after repeated losings. According to Fredrick J. Stare, M.D. and Ph.D., director, Department of Nutrition, Harvard University, researches have indicated that during the process of growing fat, damage is done to the blood vessels, particularly those of the heart.

To timetable your weight loss to from 1 to 3 pounds a week, calculate on the basis that 1 pound of fat has the fuel value of 3,500 calories.

To lose 1 pound a week cut calories by 500 a day
        2 pounds a week by   1,000 a day
        3 pounds a week by   1,500 a day

The average sedentary man requires about 2,400 calories a day for maintenance, although a physically active man needs around 3,000, and a strenuously active man even more. For a sedentary man to lose weight, therefore, he should reduce his calorie intake to from 1,400 to 2,000 a day. The average woman needs around 2,000 calories a day and can lose weight on from 1,200 to 1,500 calories a day.

Crash Diets Harmful

In general, accredited experts in weight control recommend 1,500 calories a day as the safe minimum for most dieters. Almost anyone will lose weight on that.

Few adults should go on a 1,000-calorie diet, according to clinical research at the University of Iowa Hospitals. Dr. Margaret A. Ohlson, director of the Department of Nutrition, states that a 1,000-calorie diet represents the smallest amount of calories which will provide a reasonably adequate diet without recourse to a controlled laboratory formula. Nor should any lay person attempt the use of a formula feeding unless hospitalized under guidance of a qualified physician.

Despite its lack of dramatic appeal, the pound a week loss has much in its favor. The gradualness of the loss will not upset you emotionally, cause any spectacular twist in your daily eating or endanger nutritional balance. Nor will it produce the wrinkles and scrawny neck which follow when the shrinkage of fatty tissue is faster than the elasticity of the skin over it, particularly in those middle-aged or older.

If you stick to your losing a pound a week routine, in a year you will have lost 52 pounds. You will probably not regain it. Put a tape measure around 52 pounds of fat and you will realize that it is a large order.

Painless Pound a Week Loss No Strain

Cutting out 500 calories a day from your present diet can be relatively painless. Look at these three groups of foods totaling 500 calories. Even though all food items listed are wholesome, they can be cut from your day's eating pattern without causing nutritional imbalance.

When nutritionists and physicians recommend the 1,500-calories-a-day diet, they refer to a diet whose 1,500 calories come from all the protective foods necessary to maintain bodily health. How fast you will lose on such a diet depends on your health, body structure, sex and activity.

	APPROXIMATE NUMBER OF CALORIES
1 sweet potato with 1 teaspoon butter or margarine	285
1 English muffin with butter or margarine	155
1 teaspoon jelly	30
1 teaspoon marmalade	53
	523
1 piece apple pie	290
1 doughnut	135
1 serving fruit-flavored gelatin	83
	508

COCKTAIL SNACKS

10 medium potato chips	110
3 cheese crackers	36
3 small pretzels	37
4 large ripe olives	40
4 large green olives	30
¼ cup salted peanuts	201
½ ounce Swiss cheese	50
	504

The 1,500-calorie diet (adequate for adults only) given below is recommended by the American Dietetic Association. It is flexible enough not to interfere with normal social life, will supply all the minerals, vitamins, protein and other nutrients necessary for good health, and at the same time help you lose weight.

Diet Patterns of 1,500, 1,200 and 1,800 Calories

These are based on the assumption you will take regular moderate exercise daily while following them. On them you will lose weight yet won't be hungry.

1,500-CALORIE DAILY DIET PATTERN (adequate for adults only)

1 pint whole milk

1 egg

5 ounces lean meat, poultry, fish (broiled, boiled or roasted), or cheese. May be divided between lunch and dinner. Liver once weekly.

½ cup enriched or whole-grain cereal, 1 small potato, 4 slices enriched or whole-wheat bread (See below for substitutions)

1 serving green or yellow vegetable

2 servings other vegetables (See below for vegetable choices)

1 serving citrus fruit or tomato
(4-ounce glass grapefruit or orange juice; 8-ounce glass tomato juice)

2 servings other fruit (fresh or unsweetened)

4 teaspoons butter or enriched margarine (See below for fat substitutions)

If your weekly weight loss is a little too slow on the 1,500-calorie pattern, you may want to drop it to 1,200 calories.

1,200-CALORIE DAILY DIET PATTERN (adequate for adults only)

Modify the 1,500-calorie diet by substituting skim milk or buttermilk for whole milk and omitting cereal, potato, or 1 slice of bread and 1 teaspoon fat.

On the other hand, if your weekly loss on the 1,500-calorie pattern seems a little too much for you, then add 300 calories a day.

1,800-CALORIE DAILY DIET PATTERN (adequate for adults only)

Modify the 1,500-calorie diet by adding two servings from the bread substitution list, 1 teaspoon fat and 1 ounce meat.

If you want to exchange a slice of bread for a baked potato in this pattern, do it. The plan is so flexible, many changes in specific foods can be made without upsetting the nutritional balance or calorie count.

FOR ONE SLICE OF BREAD YOU CAN SUBSTITUTE

Biscuit, roll (2-inch diameter)	1
Muffin (2-inch diameter)	1
Corn Bread (1½-inch cube)	1
Flour	2½ level tbsp.
Cereal: cooked	½ cup
dry (flake and puffed)	¾ cup
rice and grits, cooked	½ cup
Spaghetti and noodles, cooked	½ cup
Crackers: graham (2½-inch square)	2
oysterettes (½ cup)	20
saltines (2-inch square)	5
soda (2½-inch square)	3
round, thin (1½-inch diameter)	6 to 8

Vegetables: (prepared without sugar or additional
fat)

beans and peas, dried cooked (lima, navy, split, cowpeas)	½ cup
lima, fresh	½ cup
corn, sweet	⅓ cup
parsnips	⅔ cup

Potatoes: white (baked or boiled, 2-inch diameter)	1
white, mashed	½ cup
sweet or yams	¼ cup

Desserts:
1 dip or ½ cup vanilla ice cream can replace 1
slice bread and 2 teaspoons fat
1 piece angel food or sponge cake, 1½-inch cube

FAT SUBSTITUTES

You may substitute one of the following fat exchanges for 1
teaspoon of butter or margarine. Use the foods on this list only
as allowed on your meal plan. For example, if you use a teaspoon
of fat to fry an egg, give up 1 teaspoon of butter or margarine.

Butter *or* Margarine	1 teaspoon
Bacon, crisp	1 slice
Cream, light	2 tablespoons
Cream, heavy	1 tablespoon
Cream cheese	1 tablespoon
French dressing	1 tablespoon
Mayonnaise	1 teaspoon
Oil *or* Cooking fat	1 teaspoon
Peanut butter	1 teaspoon

1,500-CALORIE MENU PATTERN

Using the basic 1,500-calorie menu pattern, you can easily plan
balanced and calorie-limited menus according to your particular
tastes. Here, for example, is a sample of breakfast, lunch and
dinner for one day.

BREAKFAST

Citrus fruit *or* tomato
Egg, 1
Whole-wheat or enriched toast, 1 slice
Butter *or* Enriched margarine, 1 teaspoon
Cereal, ½ cup with milk (part of total 1 pint for the day)
Coffee

LUNCH

Lean meat *or* Meat substitute, 2 ounces
Vegetable *or* Salad
Whole-wheat or enriched bread, 2 slices
Butter *or* Enriched margarine, 1 teaspoon
Fruit
Whole milk (part of total allowed for the day)

DINNER

Lean meat *or* Meat substitute, 3 ounces
Vegetable
Potato, 1 small
Salad
Whole-wheat or enriched bread, 1 slice
Butter *or* Enriched margarine, 2 teaspoons
Fruit
Whole milk (part of total allowed for the day)

You may want to vary the kinds of protein used in these menus. This conversion table will help you.

2 ounces lean meat, 2 thin slices, 4 inches square
2 ounces meat patty, diameter 2-inch and ¾-inch thick
2 ounces whitefish, 4 inches square, ½-inch thick
2 ounces cottage cheese, ½ cup
2 ounces cheddar cheese, 2 thin slices, 4 inches square
2 ounces poultry, 1 leg or 2 slices breast or 1 thigh

Equal to one of the above:

2 eggs
4 level tablespoons peanut butter

PART II

EMOTIONAL
STABILITY
NECESSARY
FOR WEIGHT
CONTROL

CHAPTER 6

Exercise
Aids Dieter's
Stability

LET'S FACE IT. Most people who begin a weight-reduction program don't stick to it. They lose a few pounds, or maybe many pounds. But then they give up the good fight.

Why? No one quite knows all the answers. Scientists have not yet been able to discover exactly what makes people eat more food than they need. The one thing they do know is that when energy intake (calories) is greater than energy output (calories needed to maintain you at maximum performance according to age, activity, sex and build), a person puts on fat.

Their experience in obesity clinics, hospitals and group therapy convinces them that those few who do stick to their weight-control program, who accept re-education of their eating habits and learn to live happily within a calorie budget, are almost without exception emotionally well-adjusted men and women.

Emotionally stable people are usually those best adjusted to the cultural pattern of their times. In terms of food, our cultural pattern is defined as what we learned to eat at our mother's table, what our neighbors eat, what our supermarkets offer and what advertisers feature in alluring pictures. Our cultural pattern is shaped also by regional food habits and by inherited tastes.

Abundance of food in ever increasing variety is a major factor in our gastronomic cultural pattern. Not scarcity but overabundance now shapes our eating habits. Current social and economic

pressures on all of us urge us into overeating. Not just occasionally, but every day, most of us are eating more than we need.

Moderate Regular Exercise Needed

Eating too much (greater energy intake than energy output),
we have discussed. But restriction of calories, though of major
importance, is not enough by itself. Moderate and *regular*
physical exercise is necessary too.

We rarely walk any more. Furthermore, push-button homes
have reduced to a minimum the amount of physical activity
needed. In vast areas of human activity, machines and obedient
power are taking the place of flexed muscles.

However, our need for physical activity remains as constant
as it did in the time of our forefathers, because human physiology
has not changed.

Those larger waistlines, those well-tailored paunches and
heavier thighs that begin to develop after the age of thirty are
the result not only of too much good food, but also the result
of taking it too easy.

At twenty-five, we reach our optimum development. From
then on we begin to age physically. It takes fewer calories to
keep us going because the calorie cost of living normally de-
creases every year.

Although we need fewer calories, most of us go right on eating either the same amount or more, and at the same time take
less exercise. The unused calories are stored up on us as fat.

Therefore, unless we limit calories to our physical "burn-up"
needs, year by year we add unwanted pounds which can become
a health hazard.

Even though we may not eat any more than we did at twenty-
five (but most of us do), and even though we may be just as
active as we were then (an unlikely situation), we need fewer
calories to function (the calorie cost of living).

Therefore, most of us store up a few extra unused calories
every day. It is a delicious form of self-deception. Even so small
an excess as 10 to 15 unused calories a day can, over fifteen
years, add 10 to 15 pounds of body weight. (One tablespoon of

whole milk contains about 10 calories, one teaspoon of sugar around 16 calories, two large plain or stuffed green olives about 15 calories.)

Why not be honest with ourselves. Most of us eat a lot more than 10 to 15 excess calories a day. So don't be amazed at those double chins and spare tires. The fact that you are a well-satisfied victim of the easeful and prodigal cultural pattern of your time can explain why you are 10, or more, percent overweight. But it does not lessen the chances that you are endangering your health and looks.

Get Out of Your Chair More Often

Once you have passed twenty-five years, when you reach your optimum weight, and after which physiological aging begins (that is a tough fact of life to face, isn't it?) weight control becomes a definite and constant problem. There is a manageable solution: get out of your chair more often and nibble less.

If you eat a little less than you are now eating each day, and move about a little more, you will at least check your increase in weight. If you do this faithfully over a long period, you will slowly and steadily lose weight, yet at the same time be able to live in your contemporary cultural pattern. That means it is possible to lose weight (but slowly) without the usual emotional upset that results from nutritionally inadequate starvation and fad diets. Emotional upset, remember, is one of the major reasons why so many millions of dieters fall off the weight-control wagon and land right back on the fat side of the street.

Calorie control and exercise, fueled by common sense and will power, are the basic forces in any long-term weight-control program. Neither one alone can do the trick.

Exercise is an omnibus term. It can mean walking upstairs, pushing the baby carriage, whipping egg whites, sneezing, making beds, or kissing. It can also mean pounding a typewriter, standing while filing papers, delivering the office mail, lighting a cigarette, swatting a mosquito, or walking the dog. Any flexing of the muscles, great or little, is exercise, as used here, and burns up fuel, which is calories.

Restless, energetic people who seem never to stand still burn up more calories than relaxed, placid people. An impatient man who rushes across the room to switch TV channels, burns up several more calories than the fellow in the armchair, with remote control. The father who sends Johnny for his pipe burns up fewer calories than the independent parent who goes upstairs for it himself. The woman who drags her market cart home has a smaller amount of excess calories to handle than the woman who orders by phone.

A typist (weighing around 120 pounds) burns almost 88 calories an hour using a standard mechanical typewriter. But on an electric typewriter, she would burn up only about 73 calories an hour. If she types six hours a day for a five-day week, she will use up 450 calories more on the mechanical typewriter than on the electric one. In ten weeks, that will add up to 4,500 calories, the equivalent of more than a pound of body weight (allowing 3,500 calories per pound of body weight).

Energetic People Burn More Calories

Scientists have calculated that energetic people in the "white collar" brackets may burn up 66 calories an hour more than their "why not take it easy" brethren. In terms of body weight, and that is what we are discussing, this means that an energetic, nervous or physically independent man or woman burns up the equivalent of 1 pound more every seventy hours.

Exercise also means activity that involves the whole body, such as walking, swimming, dancing and tennis, etc. Small overweight persons often complain that though they exercise as regularly as their larger overweight friends, they do not lose as fast as the bigger fellows. That is because in any activity involving the whole body, the calorie use varies with the size of your body. For example, a man weighing 134 pounds walked at the rate of 3.5 miles per hour. He spent only 261 calories doing it. But a man weighing 200 pounds, walking the same distance at the same rate of speed, burned up 366 calories, or 105 calories more.

In other words, the amount of freight aboard determines the amount of fuel (calories) needed to move it. Of course, a small

person, desiring to burn up calories faster, could carry extra
pounds in a bag when he goes walking. In fact, that has been
done. A 150-pound man used about 99 calories to walk a mile.
But when he carried an extra weight of 88 pounds on his
shoulders, he burned up 142 calories walking a mile, a difference
of 43 calories.

The main fact to remember is that all forms of physical
activity have a calorie cost—the amount of calories used. The
calorie cost varies depending on the activity and, to a degree,
on the body weight of the person involved. But any physical
movement helps burn up excess calories to a large or small degree, and is therefore important in your weight control efforts.

Too many calories are not the only cause of overweight. Many
studies have proved that lack of physical activity can be a
major factor in overweight. A controlled study made in Boston
indicated that difference *in activity* between two similar groups
of high-school girls who ate the same amount of food determined
the difference between slimness and overweight. The slim girls,
who consumed as many calories as the fat girls (of the same age,
height and physical maturity), took greater part in sports and
other strenuous activities. Regular exercise therefore appeared
to help keep their weight under control.

Fit Exercise into Your Cultural Pattern

Although regular physical activity (muscle flexing) is necessary
in weight control or weight loss, it should fit into our modern
cultural pattern as do hiking, square dancing, tennis, bowling,
golf and swimming.

However, it is moderately active daily exercise that is most
important. A physically violent week end followed by five
flatulent days at the office can be harmful, increase appetite
enormously, and may even put undue strain on your heart. On
the other hand, a mile walk every day, or even a half mile, will
be more effective in your efforts at weight control than digging
up the garden over Saturday and Sunday, or ten sets of tennis
or two afternoons of sand-lot baseball with the youngsters.

The sound advice: walk, don't ride, whenever you can, may

seem startling in this motorized era. However, despite better and faster and more luxurious cars, muscles of the human body still require regular flexing. So let's take a walk.

Walk to the station from your home, walk to the PTA meeting, walk to church or to the cocktail party. Walk down a few flights of stairs in the office, get out of your taxi a few blocks from home, walk to the bank, to the dentist or that luncheon date. Get the habit of walking and you'll find it far easier to get the habit of not getting fat.

Walking a mile slowly, at the rate of two and a half miles an hour, will use about 65 to 75 calories. Walking rapidly, at the rate of four miles an hour, will use about 150 to 200 calories, according to experiments at the Harvard School of Public Health.

Therefore if you walk a mile a day in addition to your other activities: in a week, by walking slowly, you use up 455 to 525 calories; by walking more rapidly, 1,050 to 1,400 calories.

Here is a footnote to walking: for the average adult to lose a pound requires a loss of 3,500 calories. If this loss is spread over one week, it means a loss of 500 calories a day. This loss can be obtained by eating 500 calories a day less than usual, or by expending 500 calories a day more. Better yet, it can be obtained by eating from 250 to 350 calories less and exercising off 150 to 250 calories more.

Exercise Conducive to Emotional Stability

Moderate exercise every day is important, too, in keeping you emotionally stable while cutting down on your habitual intake of food. It improves muscle tone and speeds up circulation, thereby giving you a sense of well-being. This sense of well-being is very important at a time when you are denying yourself amounts of food you are used to. No matter how determined you may be to trim off fat, re-education of your appetite can be subtly upsetting at first, making you emotionally tense. Then is when you need the relaxation that walking or any other not too strenuous exercise brings.

In studying tables of calorie cost of various activities, remember that values are indicated for periods of motion only.

Note, also in some activities, such as walking, motion is constant and the expenditure uniform. But in tennis or bowling, for example, the player is in strenuous motion only part of the time.

The following tables are based on a study of food intake and energy expenditure of cadets in training, published in the *British Journal of Nutrition*.

Caloric Cost of Daily Living Activities and Sports in Men*

NORMAL ACTIVITY	CAL./MIN.	SPORT	CAL./MIN.
Standing, light activity	1.41	Football	5.04
Shower	1.84	Basketball	4.31
Dressing	1.84	Ping-pong	2.42
Making bed	2.64	Bowling	4.06
Shining shoes	2.11	Swimming	6.06
Mopping floor	2.67	Golfing	2.76
Walking indoors	1.68	Tennis	3.50
Walking outdoors	3.07	Squash	5.00
Walking upstairs	10.00	Table tennis	2.00
Walking downstairs	3.80	Badminton	1.91
Squatting	1.12	Rowing	4.00
Washing clothes	1.46	Sailing	1.30
		Dancing	2.00
		Riding	1.50
		Boxing, Sparring	5.00

* *Based on basal metabolic rate of 0.59 calories per minute per square meter of surface area.*

CHAPTER 7

Get Rid
of Tensions
Before Dieting

DESPITE ALL the books and all the advice on how to lose unwanted pounds, the record of success is discouraging. Only one
person out of four who goes on a diet and loses some pounds,
maintains that loss permanently. Seventy-five percent of dieters
abandon their weight-reduction program after a relatively short
period and regain what they have lost.

A weight-control program that will have reasonable chances
of being followed permanently, must have three objectives:

1. To reduce calorie intake to calorie expenditure.
2. To maintain nutritional balance despite limiting of calories.
3. To keep dieter emotionally stable while reducing.

Researchers in the problems of obesity now stress more and
more that relative emotional stability is essential to any lasting
weight loss. Too often the need for it is overlooked in the dieter's
panic eagerness to banish fat.

Furthermore, among scientists trying to diagnose the national
problem of obesity, there is a growing conviction that emotional
instability is one of the basic causes of overweight.

A report in *American Journal of Clinical Nutrition* on experiments at Cornell University reveals that the stable dieters, with
few or not any emotional problems, had a high degree of success
in weight reduction.

On the other hand, dieters who were tense, anxious or insecure, were less successful and gained weight during periods of stress when they used food in an attempt to find relief. Dieters who had deep-seated emotional problems failed largely to lose weight and those few who did lose weight suffered increased emotional instability.

The urge to overeat is a frequent and favored method of handling strong feeling by some people. Walter W. Hamburger, M.D., of the Department of Psychiatry of Strong Memorial Hospital and the University of Rochester School of Medicine and Dentistry, reports that certain obese patients eat when they feel blue, angry, sexually excited, apprehensive or ashamed, as though eating protected them from feeling too much.

In the *Journal of the American Dietetic Association,* he cautioned that many obese patients actually rebel against all reducing methods. Others get emotionally upset if they do reduce, and still others, while reducing, turn to substitute satisfactions such as overdrinking, oversmoking or drugs.

Dieting Can Be Harmful to Anxious People

Even though you may know you are much overweight, don't be shamed or pressured into drastic reducing unless you are sure you can maintain a reasonable amount of emotional security while doing it. Obesity is a misfortune, not a crime, remember. Reduce some of your tensions and anxieties first, then reduce your weight. Dieting to people with deep emotional problems can be harmful, especially on many of the formulae and crash diets currently popular.

Studies at the University of Pittsburgh of 400 obese middle-aged men and women between the ages of forty and sixty, the period when obesity is most prevalent and emotional tensions and responsibilities tend to increase, demonstrate the close relationship between tension and overeating. After unwanted pregnancy, death of a member of the family, or other emotional crisis, many of the women put on weight and often abandoned their diet completely.

The researches concluded that attempts at weight reduction

must be carried out with the idea of replacing the dieter's emotional need for food with some other kind of emotional support.

Therefore, if because of medical advice or the desire to look more attractive physically, you decide to go on a long-term weight-reduction program, be certain of your emotional support. Seek activities that will relax tensions while you are cutting down on food. Any activity that will take you out of yourself and enlarge your interests will make less difficult the self-discipline needed for your program.

Seek Activities That Relax Tensions

Some of the stabilizing activities suggested are working with volunteer groups in hospitals, schools, playgrounds, joining a political or literary club or musical society, hobbies such as photography or painting or stamp collecting, more intensive reading or theatergoing or participation in moderately active outdoor sports, or gardening. Any of these will help you get outside of yourself, and you will have less time for self-pity.

A diet, unless medically prescribed and supervised, that throws you to any degree outside your normal cultural pattern, is liable to be unsuccessful and short-lived because it may cause emotional upset. That is why continuing to eat with the family or with your social group is recommended. Of course you must eat less, but you will eat in general most of the same foods they do.

The two examples of 2,200-calorie one-day menus are recommended for people who hesitate to diet because of fear of emotional upset. The calories may be a little high for most women and a little low for most men. But because of the variety of foods used, the relatively low-fat content (30 percent of calories from fat), and the enjoyment possible, they, and other menus equally well-balanced nutritionally, can serve as a preliminary discipline in common-sense dieting. They were planned for that purpose by Dr. Fredrick J. Stare, chairman of the Department of Nutrition at Harvard University.

Two 2,200-Calorie One-Day Menus

Menu I (APPROXIMATELY 2,200 CALORIES)

BREAKFAST

Orange juice	½ cup
Cereal	1 cup
Milk, whole	1 cup
Sugar	1 teaspoon
Egg	
Toast	1 slice
Jam	1 tablespoon
Coffee *or* Tea	

LUNCH OR SUPPER

French onion soup	
Saltines	4
Liverwurst on rye	
Tomato, on lettuce cup	1 medium
stuffed with cottage cheese	¼ cup
Angel cake	1 piece
Coffee *or* Tea	

DINNER

Shrimp cocktail	5 shrimp
with sauce	4 tablespoons
Broiled chicken	¼ medium broiler
Rice	¾ cup
with butter	1 pat
French-style green beans,	½ cup
seasoned with thyme, green onion	
Endive, lettuce, grapefruit salad, with oil	1½ teaspoons oil
and vinegar dressing	
Rolls	2 small
Guava jelly	2 tablespoons
Fruit	
Coffee *or* Tea	

BETWEEN-MEALS SNACK (Choice of one)

Soft drink	1
Fruit juice	4-ounce average
Milk, whole	1 cup
Graham crackers	4
or	
Plain cookies	2

Menu II (APPROXIMATELY 2,200 CALORIES)

BREAKFAST

Sliced orange	
Cereal	1 cup
Milk, whole	1 cup
Sugar	1 teaspoon
Toast	1 slice
Strawberry jam	1 tablespoon
Coffee *or* Tea	

LUNCH OR SUPPER

Roast veal	3 ounces
Spaghetti	½ cup
with tomato sauce	¼ cup
Frozen peas	½ cup
Italian bread	1 slice
Jelly	1 tablespoon
Milk, whole	1 cup
Frozen peaches	½ cup
Coffee *or* Tea	

DINNER

Lean baked pork loin seasoned with mustard and Worcestershire sauce	4 ounces
Baked potato	1 medium
with sour cream and chives	1 tablespoon
Broccoli	½ cup
Lettuce Salad with vinegar	
Small roll	1

Marmalade	1 tablespoon
Lemon chiffon pie	1 serving
Coffee *or* Tea	

BETWEEN-MEALS SNACK (Choice of one)

Soft Drink	1
Fruit juice	4-ounce average
Milk, whole	1 cup
Graham crackers	4
or	
Plain crackers	2

CHAPTER 8

Crash Diets
Upset Social Pattern

LIKE GROWING up normally, growing slender, if you are fat, takes a long time. Particularly if you have been overweight for years or were stout as a child.

Any violent attack on obesity is dangerous, both physiologically and psychologically. If you doubt this, look at some of your friends who are on "crash diets," trying to lose from 7 to 15 pounds in a week. They may be taking appetite depressors, pills to speed up metabolism, or else trying to assuage self-induced hunger pangs with quarts of black coffee or by smoking incessantly, while they follow a diet of eggs and fruit juice, bananas and skim milk, dried prunes and tea or some such fantastic combination; or they may be trying to sustain life on a "fabulous formula" without advice of their doctors. Admittedly, they all do lose weight rapidly.

But what price no hips? Usually, jitters, drawn looks, irascibility and fatigue. Also, your friend most likely has become Social Enemy No. 1 by forcing all she meets to hear about her sacrifices on the altar of instant slenderness. Most physicians and nutritional researchers would diagnose her as being physically and emotionally off balance, suffering from both malnutrition and psychic shock.

How long can such drastic reducing crash diets last? Studies at obesity clinics and medical records indicate that most men and women who try to strip pounds off their bodies as they would their shirts in most cases soon return to their old eating habits and regain the fat so painfully lost.

Underlying any practical long-term reduction routine must be acceptance of the fact we all live in the world together. It just is not true that nobody loves a fat man. Or woman. Overweight people have family, relatives and friends just like their leaner counterparts on the bathroom scales. The demands of domestic and communal life fall on the unreduced and the reduced alike. Therefore any diet that banishes the dieter to social isolation or commits him to a hermit's cell, cannot be long endured.

Avoid Social Isolation While Reducing

To maintain emotional stability while reducing, eating with the family is urged by both psychiatrists and dietitians. Unless the dieter can stay reasonably within the accustomed cultural and family pattern, he is liable to become depressed and tempted to chuck the diet.

Of course you will eat less. Even so, you will eat the same familiar foods the average meal planner buys in her market. No matter how many pounds you decide to lose, you need the same kinds of food and in the same variety that non-dieting members of the family need. But remember, in smaller quantities.

At the University of California School of Public Health in Berkeley, nutritionists have experimented with family menus that make it practical for the special dieter in the home to draw up his chair and enjoy his meals with the family. They have found that when the dieter is a member of the social group instead of an isolated individual, he is saved from the depression that so often destroys his determination to stick to his weight-loss program.

Before a dieter joins the family table, however, they remind him that the calorie count of different foods depends on the relative amounts of fat, sugar, starch, protein, or water or fiber they contain. Water and fiber, present in large amounts in vegetables and to a lesser degree in fruits, provide no calories.

For this reason, celery, asparagus, cabbage, eggplant, radishes, tomatoes, summer squash, lettuce greens and other leafy vegetables add virtually no calories to the dieter's daily total. Therefore, they may be eaten in unrestricted amounts in reduction diets.

On the other hand, foods containing relatively little water and

Menus for the Family with a Dieter

APPROXIMATELY 1,500 CALORIES FOR DIETER

APPROXIMATELY 2,500 CALORIES FOR RELATIVELY ACTIVE ADULT MALES AND 11-YEAR-OLD GIRLS

APPROXIMATELY 3,600 CALORIES FOR 17-YEAR-OLD BOYS AND VERY ACTIVE ADULTS

Breakfast

1,500 Calories

Melon or Grapefruit
Fluffy herb omelet (1-egg portion) cooked in 1 teaspoon butter
1 slice whole-wheat toast with 1 teaspoon butter or 2 teaspoons jelly

Coffee (black)

2,500 Calories

Melon or Grapefruit
Fluffy herb omelet (1-egg portion) cooked in butter
2 slices whole-wheat toast with butter
Jelly
2 strips bacon
1 glass whole milk for girl
Coffee for adult

3,600 Calories

Melon or Grapefruit
Fluffy herb omelet (1-egg portion) cooked in butter
3 slices whole-wheat toast with butter
Jelly
4 strips bacon
1 glass whole milk

Lunch

1,500 Calories

Tomato bouillon (no calories in fat-free bouillon)
Open-faced sandwich with lettuce, 1-ounce meat, 1 teaspoon mayonnaise
Celery, carrot, green pepper sticks
1 glass milk, non-fat
½ cup plain ice cream

2,500 Calories

Tomato bouillon
Meat sandwich with lettuce and mayonnaise
Vegetable sticks
1 glass whole milk
Ice cream with topping if desired

3,600 Calories

Tomato bouillon
2 sandwiches with lettuce and mayonnaise
Vegetable sticks
1 glass whole milk
Ice cream with topping if desired

51

After-School or Evening Snack

1 portion fresh fruit

Fresh fruit

Fresh fruit, sandwich
1 glass milk

Dinner

Oven-broiled chicken paprika (wrapped in foil and cooked without fat added)
Baked white potato with 1 teaspoon butter and ¾ cup hot milk
Frozen or fresh broccoli (no added butter) with lemon wedge
Mixed vegetable salad herb vinegar dressing
Frozen strawberries (unsweetened)
1 glass milk, non-fat (8 ounces)

Oven-broiled chicken (brushed with butter)
Baked sweet potato with butter
Broccoli
Mixed vegetable salad
French dressing
1 roll and butter
Strawberry shortcake
Whole milk

Oven-broiled chicken (brushed with butter) (2 servings)
Baked sweet potatoes with butter
Broccoli
Mixed vegetable salad
French dressing
2 rolls and butter
Strawberry shortcake
Whole milk

NOTE: *For more menus for families with dieters, see pages 85-99.*

fiber, such as breads and cereals, are higher in calories, particularly so if they contain fat as well as starch and protein.

As to the calorie value of sugar, starch and protein, they are alike. But fats contain much more, slightly more than twice as many as sugars, starches and protein. That is why moderation in use of fats is wise for the reducer.

The preceding "Menus for the Family with a Dieter" make a place at the table for the dieter on 1,500 calories a day, who will eat the same foods as the non-dieting members of the family but in smaller amounts. No special "natural" or "health" foods are required. All the ingredients come from the well-stocked American supermarket.

PART III

SUCCESSFUL
REDUCING
DIETS USE
FAMILIAR
FOODS

CHAPTER 9

Bread Permitted
in Reducing Diets

RESEARCH scientists in obesity, and dietitians and psychiatrists in obesity clinics know from thousands of case histories that any diet which too drastically and too suddenly tries to change life-long and traditionally ingrained eating habits is headed for failure.

That is why "crash diets" are a waste of time. They are physically brutal, nutritionally reckless and psychologically ruthless. Although they may lop off fat with a butcher's speed, they function on the principle of semistarvation.

To lose weight, of course, you must reduce your calorie intake. But that does not mean you have to banish any single food from your reducing diet. All good foods are good, remember, even though some may contain more calories than others. But it's the total amount of calories in your entire day's meals more than the number of calories in any single food that will determine the rate of weight loss.

Such foods as potatoes, bread, sugar and ice cream, etc., are good foods. If they are a deeply entrenched part of your cultural pattern and you enjoy them, they can be fitted into your calorie budget. Even on a 1,500-calorie diet, there is nothing you cannot eat some of the time. Not in accustomed quantities and with no seconds, however. Nor as regularly as you have been eating them. Therefore, for the sake of wide variety in your reducing menus, and to prevent feeling "deprived," as well as for their wholesomeness, include them in your general plan.

Bread Often Emotionally Necessary

To many people, bread is the gastronomical symbol of security. Emotionally (not nutritionally) they feel insecure without it. For those people, therefore, some bread in reducing menus is essential to maintain the psychological balance without which they will not be able to stick to a long-term program.

Reporting on her experience as a dietitian in an army hospital in the South Pacific during World War II, Dr. Martha F. Trulson, associate professor of nutrition at Harvard University, reports that most soldiers demand bread no matter how much other food there is in the meal. Once when the supply was shut off for several days, even though they were adequately fed, both nutritionally and in quantity, the men were restless without their bread.

To many Americans of foreign ancestry, breads of their parents' national origin have been an essential, and often a very large, part of their daily food. Suddenly to be diverted from a lifelong habit associated with family security would almost inevitably throw them off emotional balance. As children we learned in school, in copy books, and at home, that bread is the staff of life, and our parents never objected when we wolfed a slice of bread with butter and jam after school. All these experiences have given bread a favorable association value. To tell an overweight man or woman who has always regarded bread as part of a normal pattern of living that it has no place in a reducing diet would be almost as upsetting as to say "Forget about mother love—it is fattening."

Fit Bread into Your Calorie Budget

So if you cannot be happy without a slice of bread every now and then, either because you enjoy the taste or are emotionally attached to it, enjoy it in good conscience. An average slice of American bread is about 63 to 70 calories, a pat (level teaspoon) of butter about 45 calories. But you must fit those 108 calories into your 1,500-calorie pattern without upsetting its nutritional balance.

Remember that bread, like charity, has many forms: white, whole-wheat, rye, protein, French and Italian, plus rolls of many types. Their calorie content differs.

The scientifically planned 1,500-calorie (approximately) diet that follows will keep any bread lover reasonably happy. It includes coffee cake with nuts and icing, is nutritionally balanced and could be enjoyed by your non-dieting family and friends.

Bread-Eater's 1,500-Calorie Diet

BREAKFAST

Grapefruit	½ medium
Coffee cake with nuts and icing	4½-inch diameter
Crisp bacon	1 slice
Scrambled egg (cooked with 1 tablespoon whole milk and 2 teaspoons fat)	1
Coffee *or* Tea	
Sugar	1 teaspoon

LUNCH

Chicken noodle soup	1 cup
Bologna sandwich: bread	2 slices
bologna	2 slices
mustard	
Milk, non-fat	8 ounces

DINNER

Baked sole (baked in milk)	3 ounces
Carrots	1 cup
Parsley potato	1 small
1 teaspoon fat	
Lettuce with tangerine section,	1
cottage cheese	½ cup
Fresh fruit gelatin	
Coffee *or* Tea	

SNACKS

Tomato juice	4 ounces
Milk, non-fat	8 ounces

CHAPTER 10

Beef Included
in Reducing Diets

TODAY, a thick juicy steak is the American symbol of success. Overweight or not, most men and women dream of eating as much of it as they can afford.

On the tested theory that a continuing weight-control program must adjust to the dieter's cultural program, beef belongs in a nutritionally balanced reducing diet. Not only is it one of the best sources of protein, but its satiety value to most men and women is very high.

The average domestic serving of beef is ⅓ pound without bone. However, restaurant servings are generally larger, and in many homes men particularly demand at least ½ pound.

Many people consider the fat surrounding steaks and roast beef highly delicious and want it left on their meat. Of course, the calorie count on such meat is higher than on cuts with all visible fat trimmed off. Therefore, in determining the number of calories in the meat in your diet, be sure you base your figures on whether it is trimmed or not and also whether you use the customary ⅓-pound (5⅓ ounces) or the ½-pound (8 ounces) serving.

Trim Off Visible Fat to Reduce Calories

Top grade beef, the kind most people want, is high in calories because most tender cuts are the fattest. Trimming off the visible fat can reduce some of the calories, but the tender cuts are heavily marbled with fat and this fat cannot be trimmed off. Therefore, the dieter, if he needs beef to feel secure and well fed, must recognize the higher calorie count of the top grades of beef and fit those calories into his balanced 1,500-calorie diet. It can be done.

For example, ½ pound of untrimmed boneless Porterhouse contains approximately 675 calories. So does ½ pound filet mignon. A 3-ounce slice (3x2½x¼-inch) of untrimmed roast, has about 300 calories, and ¼ pound of hamburg (with much of the fat left in), about 265 calories.

However, if all visible fat had been trimmed from these same cuts and servings were smaller, the calorie count per serving would be much lower. For example, 3 ounces of lean and marbled Porterhouse would be only 215 calories, and 3 ounces of lean and marbled tenderloin only 200, as against 675 calories for ½ pound untrimmed.

An occasional juicy steak or a few slices of well-marbled rib roast, like any other good food at your market, belong in the beef lover's long-term reducing diet. But not too often. On other days, you should use lower-fat proteins such as chicken, turkey, fish or seafood or veal in order to keep down your average percentage of calories from fat. The younger the animal, the less fat, and consequently fewer calories, will it carry. Leaner cuts of beef can be used too. But with these other proteins, as with the top-grade beef cuts, keep the proportion of green and yellow vegetables and fruit, including some citrus, high.

The following "Steak-Eater's 1,500-Calorie Diet," prepared by the Department of Nutrition at Harvard University, is one example of how beef can be included in a reducing diet.*

Steak-Eater's 1,500-Calorie Diet

BREAKFAST

Tomato juice	4 ounces
Poached egg	1
Toast	1 slice
Coffee *or* Tea	
Sugar	1 teaspoon

* NOTE: *For other diet plans including liberal amounts of beef, see pages 146-151.*

LUNCH

Crabmeat sandwich *or* tuna, water-packed

crabmeat *or* tuna	3 tablespoons
chopped celery	1 tablespoon
prepared salad dressing	1 tablespoon
whole-wheat bread	2 slices
Medium apple	
Milk, non-fat	8 ounces

DINNER

Filet mignon or boneless sirloin with mushrooms	½ pound
French fried potatoes	8 pieces
Snap beans	1 serving
Lettuce and tomato with lemon	
Coffee *or* Tea	

SNACKS

Graham crackers	2
Milk, non-fat	8 ounces

The following nutritionally balanced dinner menus can be used in a 1,400- to 1,500-calorie diet. They will help the person who finds meat essential to a feeling of satiety to get enjoyment from his meals while he is losing pounds and learning to select food within a better nutritional pattern.

If a moderate slice of bread is included in each dinner menu, increase the total calories by 65. Subtract the total calories for dinner from the day's allowance of 1,500 and divide the remainder between breakfast and lunch.

1. Blade pot roast (4 ounces); green beans (½ cup); butter or margarine (1 pat); peach (½ cup); milk, non-fat (1 cup); coffee or tea, if desired. (605 calories)
2. Tomato juice (½ cup); baked ham (4 ounces); spinach (½ cup); butter or margarine (1 pat); carrot sticks (½ carrot); milk, non-fat (1 cup); coffee or tea, if desired. (432 calories)
3. Roast leg of lamb (4 ounces); carrots (½ cup); butter or margarine (1 pat); cabbage-pineapple salad (½ cup); milk, non-fat (1 cup); coffee or tea, if desired. (429 calories)

4. Smoked shoulder butt (4 ounces); cabbage (½ cup); butter or margarine (1 pat); grapefruit sections (½ cup); milk, non-fat (1 cup); coffee or tea, if desired. (578 calories)

5. Ground beef patty (4 ounces); cauliflower (½ cup); butter or margarine (1 pat); vanilla ice cream (¼ pint); milk, non-fat (1 cup); coffee or tea, if desired. (579 calories)

6. Tomato juice (½ cup); roast beef (4 ounces); wax beans (½ cup); butter or margarine (1 pat); celery sticks; milk, non-fat (1 cup); coffee or tea, if desired. (511 calories)

7. Roast turkey or roast pork loin (4 ounces); carrots (½ cup); butter or margarine (1 pat); sliced tomato (1 small); mayonnaise (1 tablespoon); milk, non-fat (1 cup); coffee or tea, if desired. (545 calories)

CHAPTER 11

Dieter Can Have
a Baked Potato

WHAT COULD be more American than a big baked potato with a lump of butter on it? You'd give anything for one. But you are on a 1,500-calorie-a-day diet. So how do you get around that baked potato problem?

Very simply. You eat it.

In the first place, potatoes are nutritious food and important in the cultural pattern of most people. Like bread, they are commonly a symbol of security. Without them, many dieters feel deprived. Therefore, in a sound reducing diet that can be followed consistently for a long term, potatoes should be included occasionally. They can be used as a bread exchange any time.

Actually, they are not high in calories. A medium potato has about 100 calories, a large baker type may run up to 200. Add a teaspoon of butter to a medium potato and the total runs up to 145. However, considering the nutritive and psychological value of a baked or boiled potato in the balanced reducing diet, those calories will be well spent.

However, don't allow the inclusion of a potato in your menu plan to upset the nutritional balance of your total daily calories.

The two sample 1,500-calorie-a-day diets below include potatoes without distorting the nutritional balance. Use them as a guide in planning your diets.

Two Sample 1,500-Calorie Diets

Sample 1. 1,500-Calorie Diet

BREAKFAST

Medium grapefruit	½
Corn flakes	¾ cup
Whole milk	8 ounces
Toast	1 slice
Marmalade	1 tablespoon
Coffee *or* Tea	
Sugar	1 teaspoon

LUNCH

Bouillon (from cubes)	
Cheese crackers	4
Salad julienne	
hard-cooked egg	½
shredded boiled ham	1 ounce
shredded cheese	½ ounce
tomato, lettuce, celery	
vinegar, seasonings	
Grapes	1 small bunch
Tea	

DINNER

Baked potato	1 medium
Sour cream (commercial)	2 tablespoons
Baked crab and shrimp	Moderate serving
Asparagus, lemon juice	(4 ounces)
Tossed salad, vinegar	
Coffee *or* Tea	

SNACKS

Tangerines	1 large or 2 small
Milk, non-fat	8 ounces

Sample 2. 1,500-Calorie Diet

SUNDAY BRUNCH

Orange juice	4 ounces
Waffle (5½-inch square)	1
Maple syrup	3 tablespoons
Butter	1 pat
Coffee *or* Tea	
Sugar	1 teaspoon

DINNER

Roast chicken	3 slices
Dressing	¼ cup
Mashed potatoes (made with milk and fat)	½ cup
Brussels sprouts with lemon	½ cup
Lettuce, celery, radish salad with vinegar	
Sherbet	½ cup

BEDTIME

Dry cereal	1 cup
Milk, non-fat	8 ounces
Sugar	1 teaspoon

SNACKS

Grapefruit	½
Milk, non-fat	8 ounces

Include Macaroni, Noodles and Rice Sometimes

Macaroni and noodles and other macaroni products are good foods too. They should be included occasionally in diets if the dieter is so accustomed to them that their absence might discourage him from sticking to his long-term diet.

But spaghetti products, particularly with cheese or Italian sauce, pile up the calories. For example, one cup of macaroni products, plain-cooked, has about 140 calories. Sauces with cheese, fat, tomato sauce and vegetables add many more. Therefore, on days when you indulge in a dish of your favorite spaghetti with Italian sauce, cut out some other high-calorie food to keep the day's total calories in line. However, there must be necessary servings of vegetables and fruits and some extra protein in the day's balanced diet, no matter how low your calorie budget.

There are several brands of low-calorie noodles on the market. If they taste right to you, use them.

Rice is another carbohydrate essential to dieters in certain areas of the country. Include it, too, in your balanced diets if rice is a symbol of normal living to you. There are about 70 calories in ½ cup cooked.

Although you may have been told by the unknowing that potatoes, spaghetti products and rice, as well as soup, must be banished from any reducing diet, you now see why they, like all other good foods, can be incorporated into any balanced low-calorie diet. Used in moderation, they often help the dieter's feeling of security and supply enjoyment.

Soup Important to Some Dieters

If you grew up in a household where soup was an important part of the daily family dinner, you may feel cheated without it. Feeling cheated is no spur to continuing your diet. Therefore, if soup is an ingrained part of your cultural pattern, you can enjoy a bowl now and then and still stick to your diet.

For cream soups, use your daily allotment of milk. Chill your chicken soup and skim off fat before heating. Clear beef consommé is excellent for a snack. In ¾ cup there are only 35 calories. That is very few, considering the comfort soup gives.*

* NOTE: *For 1,500-calorie diets using soups, see pages 158-168.*

CHAPTER 12

Sweets Get
Limited Space
in Diets

THE UNITED STATES is a sweet-tooth country. Although the right to have apple pie or a slice of chocolate cake is not guaranteed by the Constitution, most Americans assume it is. To millions, desserts are a necessary part of any meal, and sugar a factor in our cultural pattern. The dread of living without dessert, some candy and a little sugar in the breakfast coffee, keeps many overweight people from going on a diet.

Nutritionally sound diets for permanent weight control are flexible enough to include some sugar. They are based on psychological as well as calorie values, and so planned that the dieter will enjoy his meals even though his customary number of calories is cut by as much as 500 to 1,000 a day. They admit sugar-sweetened dishes occasionally for two reasons: our contemporary cultural pattern is liberally sweetened; it is the number of calories you eat in a day, not the number of calories in any particular food, that tip the scales either for or against you.

Actually, despite its unjustified bad name and the almost childish moral indignation some zealots feel against it, sugar is not a heavy-calorie food. One teaspoon has about 16 calories. Fats, such as butter, margarine and cooking oils, have more than twice as many calories per gram. Just 3 level teaspoons of any of the familiar cooking oils contain as many calories as 6 teaspoons of sugar. Refined sugar also has the same amount of calories per gram as good protein. It can be a "shot in the arm" when extra quick energy is demanded. And the sweetness of sugar is by many regarded as a benign factor in the good life, making their meals more satisfying.

Diet Can Include Some Sweets

Within reasonable limits, therefore, a sound diet adjusted to our cultural pattern, finds a modest place for cake and ice cream, pie and pudding and sugar, and even a piece of candy now and then. It does not necessarily recommend them for a 1,500-calorie diet. It does face the fact that they are not only good foods in varying degree, but also frequently essential to the stability of many dieters and therefore must be included occasionally.

Artificial, or non-nutritive, sweeteners, such as saccharin and Sucaryl, contain no calories and have no food value. They give a calorie-free sweet flavor and are harmless. They are used to sweeten foods and many soft drinks as well as desserts.

However, their use may trap you into fattening self-deception. Just because your coffee and tea and other beverages, as well as cakes and pies, are sweetened by non-caloric artificial sweeteners, does not mean that you are free to indulge in other non-sweet but high-calorie foods not permitted in your particular diet.

For example you may use an artificial sweetener in your coffee instead of a teaspoon of sugar, thereby saving 16 calories, and drink a bottle of no-calorie beverage instead of a sugar-sweetened one, thereby saving about 75 calories. But that doesn't mean you have done your dieting for the day and are free to eat another slice of cake in which there are calories from fat, eggs and flour and milk and maybe chocolate and nuts.

Artificial Sweets Do Not Reduce Calories Drastically

A controlled test of the effect on weight of the use of sugar by one group, and artificial sweeteners by another but matched group, of older men and women, revealed that the weight changes in the two groups were about the same. The evidence indicated in this test that the long-term use of artificial sweeteners had little, or no more, effect in weight loss over a period of time than did the use of sugar by the control group. The comparison was made by averages, however, not by individuals.

The two following 1,500-calorie diets are for your dessert days. Although apple pie à la mode and a teaspoon of sugar in coffee are given in one menu, and a cup of cocoa and a slice of angel food in the other, the nutritional balance for the two days is maintained and the calorie limit adhered to.

Two Sample Diets Including Desserts

Dessert Diet No. 1—1,500 Calories

BREAKFAST

Pineapple juice (unsweetened)	½ cup
Oatmeal	½ cup
Milk, non-fat	8 ounces
Coffee *or* Tea	
Sugar	1 teaspoon

LUNCH

Jellied consommé	
Cottage cheese	½ cup
with orange and grapefruit sections	1 cup
lettuce	
Toast	1 slice
Butter	1 pat

DINNER

Raw oysters with sauce	6
Roast veal	2 slices
Boiled onions	½ cup
Spinach with lemon juice	
Endive salad with vinegar *or* lemon juice	
Apple pie	1 moderate slice
Ice cream	¼ pint

SNACKS

Cola	6 ounces
Milk, non-fat	8 ounces

Dessert Diet No. 2—1,500 Calories

BREAKFAST

Orange juice	½ cup
Soft-cooked egg	1
Rye toast	1 slice
Jelly	1 tablespoon
Cocoa (made with milk, non-fat)	6 ounces

LUNCH

Canned split-pea soup	1 cup
with chopped ham	½ ounce
butter *or* fat	1 teaspoon
Toast as croutons	½ slice
Molded unflavored gelatin with sugar, cabbage, lemon juice	
Popover	1 average
Strawberry jam	1 tablespoon
Coffee *or* Tea	

DINNER

Chicken Cacciatore breast browned in fat with tomato sauce	4 ounces
Fresh snap beans, no fat	
Small riced potatoes	2
Lettuce wedge, vinegar	
Angel cake	1 average slice
Coffee *or* Tea	

SNACK

Milk, non-fat	8 ounces

CHAPTER 13

Cocktails
Permitted
in Some
Diets

THE COCKTAIL hour is the dieter's greatest hazard. The first drink, like the first kiss, usually leads to more. The first snack, too, casts a come-hither look at the second and the second often does the same to the third. Whatever else may happen, you are sure of one thing—*calories*.

Nevertheless, the cocktail hour, or a drink or two before or after dinner, has become an established part of the American way of living in many areas of the country. Therefore, it must be taken into consideration in any long-term weight-reduction program geared to our contemporary cultural pattern.

If a dieter has been accustomed to one or two drinks a day for many years and regards them as a normal part of his way of life, many students of obesity problems would hesitate to banish alcohol completely from his long-term program. They believe that to deprive him abruptly of what has been a socially acceptable and relaxing part of his routine might threaten his emotional balance at a time when he is undergoing diet discipline.

This is the opinion of many obesity therapists and clinical dietitians. The statement on the subject by Robert E. Shank, M.D., professor of preventive medicine at Washington University School of Medicine, St. Louis, is representative.

Clinicians have long known, and carefully undertaken investigations have established the fact, that many persons who become obese are importantly motivated by problems of insecurity. As a group they may, therefore, also be likely to find enjoyment and satisfaction in occasional or sometimes frequent use of alcoholic beverages. The effects produced by alcohol are those which can bring about important reductions of personal tensions. Therefore, it can be considered that there is real purpose to encourage or certainly not to discourage the use of such materials by obese persons who may have feelings of insecurity.

Dr. Shank warned, nevertheless, that it should not be forgotten that all such beverages contribute calories which must be counted in the daily calorie budget. When you are on a 1,200- or 1,500-calorie diet, more than a limited amount of alcohol cannot be included without crowding out foods of greater nutritional value.

Count Alcohol Calories by Ounce and Proof

In general, the way to count calories in whisky, gin and other hard liquors is this: per ounce per proof equals calories. For example, 1 ounce of 86-proof Scotch contains 86 calories, 1 ounce of 100-proof bourbon contains 100 calories and an ounce of 90-proof gin contains 90 calories. If you use ginger ale, cola, vermouth, etc. in mixing, the calories in the mixer must be added to the total in your drink.

An 8-ounce glass of beer generally contains about 104 calories, according to the Brewers Testing Laboratory. Ale has slightly more, so have foreign beers. Generally, 3 ounces of red wine contain around 70 calories; the same amount of white wine, about 80. Two ounces of sherry has about 84. Of course, dry wine has fewer calories than sweet.

If you take 300 of your 1,500 calories from alcohol (that's 20 percent), you run the risk of upsetting your nutritional balance. To help offset this danger, make certain the food you eat every day includes some from each of these categories: milk; meat; fish; poultry; cheese or eggs; bread and cereals; green and leafy vegetables; fruits, including citrus; and reasonable amounts of fats.

Also, cut down on those tempting camp followers of the cocktail party—canapés and hors d'oeuvres. That is one way to compensate for these 300 calories (or less) from your 1,500 calories. For example, a 1½-inch cube of cheddar cheese has 110 calories, 8 large potato chips have 100 and 10 peanuts 50. Turn to the tray of celery, endive spears, radishes, raw carrots and cucumber sticks instead. They are comfortably low in calories.

Another way to compensate for these alcohol calories is to increase your regular and mild daily exercise. You might walk to the cocktail party and then walk home. The sooner you start back the better.

Two Cocktails Have Same Calories as Rich Dessert

Although from a nutritional point of view, he does not recommend alcohol to dieters, Dr. Stare recognizes the obvious fact of life that some overweight men and women accustomed to social drinking will refuse to go on a diet unless they can have their habitual drink or two. He reminds them that two drinks supply about the same number of calories as a rich dessert or a good serving of meat. Therefore, cut out the dessert, not the meat, because meat supplies more protein necessary for nutritional balance.

However, as his co-worker, Dr. Martha F. Trulson, points out, alcoholic drinks and desserts are not nutritionally the same, even though they tend to be calorically the same. Most desserts contain flour, fruit, eggs and milk, all rich in nutrients, whereas alcohol contains none, only calories. Although a believer in the need to adjust weight-reduction programs to the cultural pattern, she does not recommend that obese persons take up drinking. They have enough problems. However, she and others, even though they do not recommend it from a nutritional standpoint, realize that a person on a 1,500-calorie diet who is convinced he cannot stick to it for any time without his drink or two must be given a program which allows for the calories in alcohol. To help such dieters learn how to maintain nutritional balance despite their

customary two martinis, etc., Dr. Trulson suggests the following
sample one-day menu of 1,500 calories.

Sample One-Day Menu—1,500 Calories

BREAKFAST

Grape juice	4 ounces
Small shredded wheat	1
Non-fat milk	8 ounces
Toast	1 slice
Marmalade	1 tablespoon
Coffee	
Sugar	1 teaspoon

LUNCH

Tomato soup (canned condensed, with water)	1 cup
Hot dog with bun and relish	1
Coffee *or* Tea	

DINNER

Dry martinis	2
Barbecued chicken	4 ounces
Zucchini squash	½ cup
Peas and mushrooms	½ cup
Celery	3 stalks
Parkerhouse roll	1
Coffee *or* Tea	

SNACKS

Tomato juice	4 ounces
Non-fat milk	8 ounces

Don't Upset Nutritional Balance with Cocktails

Using a 1,500-calorie diet as base, the American Dietetic Association suggests the following method of including 2 drinks
without upsetting the nutritional balance:

FOR THE DAY

Whole milk	1 pint
Meat, fish, fowl, eggs, hard cheese	6 ounces
Breads, cereals, noodles, potatoes, etc.	6 servings
Vegetables	3 servings
Fruits	3 servings
Fat	4 teaspoons

From the above diet pattern, omit 1 average slice of bread or serving of cereal (70 calories), 1 teaspoon of butter (45 calories) and substitute skim milk for whole milk (saving 170 calories). By cutting out these items, the dieter will not upset the nutritional balance but will have a credit of 285 calories to invest in liquid forms of emotional relaxation.

If you must have your 2 drinks a day while trying to reduce, use plain or carbonated water instead of ginger ale, cola, and other sweet mixers which add calories. Also, ask for a highball rather than "on the rocks." Your allotted alcohol will last longer. Another practical hint on how to prolong your cocktail hour is to serve your martinis accompanied by a tall glass of ice water and sip from each alternately. The result, in the words of Keats, will be "linked sweetness long drawn out."

The final decision, however, whether or not you can have your customary drinks and still stay within your 1,500-calorie reducing diet rests with your bathroom scales. Weigh yourself every day at the same time and under the same conditions. The scales won't lie because they are always clear-headed.

You will note on pages 163, 165, and 168 that there are menus which include drinks.

PART IV

SOUND
NUTRITION
BLOCKS
OVERWEIGHT

CHAPTER 14

Teach
Children
Not to
Get Fat

SOME of our brightest men and women are fat. This massive evidence should prove that intelligence alone will not cause anyone to lose weight. Intelligence is, however, one of the basic requirements of any sound long-term weight-control program.

Obesity is the result of eating more calories than the body needs to function. Nevertheless, the underlying causes of our persistently excessive appetites are not yet understood by scientists. They do know that the causes are very complex and probably involve heredity, psychological, and environmental (cultural pattern) factors.

Whatever the factors are, they often seem stronger than intelligence. Most overweight people are well aware of the relationship between obesity and hypertension, heart diseases, diabetes, gall bladder disease, as well as the higher death rate. Yet they find it difficult, in many cases impossible, to control their appetites.

Most overweight people acquired the habit of overeating early in life. In fact, many of us were little gluttons before we were out of diapers. As all clinicians in obesity report, the longer a person has been overweight, the more difficult it is for him to trim down to his desirable weight.

However, although there is as yet no complete scientific agreement on the causes of obesity, there is complete agreement on the need to prevent it. They insist that it is far more important, both from health and social considerations, to teach young children the habit of not getting fat than it is to teach them the habit of brushing their teeth regularly.

The catch in teaching young children the habit of not getting fat is basically one of educating the mother to good meal planning. In spite of the doctor's advice, many mothers still cling to the superstition that a plump, overfed baby is a healthy baby, that to be big is the same as to be strong and healthy.

Young Children Often Forced to Overeat

Therefore, because of ignorance, or overprotectiveness or emotionalism, mothers habitually put more food before small children than they need, and then insist or threaten or cajole until it is eaten. Also, many an unneeded bottle has been stuck in baby's mouth for no better reason than to keep him from crying.

A recent summary of scientific studies of the nutrition of infants and children, published in *Nutrition Reviews*, warns that modern mothers are constantly being reminded by advertisers of the concept that bigger babies are better babies, which is but one manifestation of a frame of mind which pervades our culture.

The summary, prepared by Gilbert B. Forbes, M.D., of the Department of Pediatrics of the University of Rochester School of Medicine and Dentistry, indicates that overdoses of vitamins and too much food for infants can be as serious a medical problem as underfeeding, and that overnutrition may actually become a curse to American children.

Research shows that most fat children and adults were not overweight at birth, even though born to fat parents. They grew fat, in most cases, because as infants they were taught and encouraged to eat more calories than they needed. Either their mothers did not restrain the uninformed urge to overfeed them, or else their parents, being "big eaters," set the example of overeating while the imitative youngsters were still in their high chairs.

This habit can result—and usually does—in teen-age and adult obesity. It can result, too, in adult desperation, because overweight in a man or woman who was fat as a child is the hardest to overcome.

Overweight in teen-agers can produce serious consequences. They are handicapped both physically and emotionally. Young women want to be beautiful and attractive to men, young men to be muscular and attractive to women. But excess fat on their growing bodies defeats them. Often it results in emotional frustration. It indicates they may be fat when they're adults, also. That is why prevention of overweight in boys and girls in their school years is so important in the lifelong battle against obesity.

W. H. Sebrell, Jr., M.D., director of the Institute of Nutrition Sciences at Columbia University, believes the answer to this problem is to establish in young children correct eating habits that will last all their lives.

He urges mothers to restrain the urge to serve fancy, high-calorie "yummy" dishes to their children, and instead, to use their talents in preparing highly nutritive dishes so attractively that acquiring good eating habits gets to be "doing what comes naturally."

Teen-agers Need Lots of Right Kinds of Food

This outstanding researcher in nutrition, with long experience in the eating habits of children and teen-agers, explains that "Growing girls and boys do need large amounts of food, of course. But that means large amounts of the right kinds of food appetizingly served, foods that provide essential nutrition on which they can grow healthy, strong and attractive. If a grammar or high school boy or girl is getting fat, there are ways to control weight without retarding normal physical growth. Fatness is not the same thing as large bones and developed muscles. The healthy growing child should get heavier every year—heavier but not fatter."

How many calories a day does the average teen-age girl or boy need? The 1958 report of the Food and Nutrition Board of the National Research Council, recommends these as the best average figures:

Children 1 to 3, approximately 1,300 calories
          4 to 6, approximately 1,700 calories
          7 to 9, approximately 2,100 calories
          10 to 12, approximately 2,500 calories
A boy 13 to 15, approximately 3,100 calories
A boy 16 to 19, approximately 3,600 calories
A girl 13 to 15, approximately 2,600 calories
But less for a girl 16 to 19—only about 2,400 calories
   (This is because girls mature physically more rapidly than
   boys.)

Food, not starvation, is the basis of all modern scientific reducing and weight-control diets. Therefore, it is imperative that
teen-agers, as well as adults, understand the four basic food
groups on which balanced diets are built. This nutritional knowledge is far more important to their social life, not to mention
their health, than the newest rock-and-roll records. Musical
evaluation aside, rock-and-roll and other forms of dancing do
contribute to the obese teen-ager's welfare. It is an occasion for
exercise. Flexing of the muscles, whether of shoulder, hip or knee,
burns up calories and improves circulation. Fat teen-agers are,
as a rule, physically lethargic, spending more time at the school
snack bar than in the gym or swimming pool.

Of course, teen-agers need a large supply of calories. But those
calories must come from the four basic food groups:

1. *Meat Group:* Two or more servings every day of beef, veal,
   lamb, pork, variety meats (liver, heart, kidney), poultry and
   eggs, fish and shellfish. As alternates: dry beans and peas,
   lentils, nuts, peanut butter. These provide protein for growth,
   iron and B vitamins.

2. *Milk Group:* Fluid, whole, evaporated, skim, non-fat dry milk,
   or buttermilk. Also cheese (cottage, cream, cheddar type).
   And ice cream. Dr. Sebrell believes teen-agers eat better with
   no more than two glasses of milk a day, although some nutritionists recommend a quart. For fat teen-agers he suggests
   non-fat dry milk or skim milk, explaining that the protein,
   calcium and vitamin B-a of milk make it important for most
   growing youngsters.

3. *Vegetable-Fruit Group:* Four or more servings a day of fruits
   and vegetables with at least one serving from orange or
   orange juice, grapefruit or grapefruit juice, which provide
   the essential vitamin C. The more dark green and yellow
   vegetables the better.
4. *Bread and Cereal Group:* Four or more servings of whole
   grain or enriched or restored cereals including breads, cooked
   or ready-to-eat cereals, macaroni, rice, noodles. These foods
   provide food energy, plus liberal amounts of protein, iron
   and several B vitamins.

It is normal for teen-agers to eat enormous amounts of food.
They have great need for calories at this actively growing period.
The major problem in leading them into correct eating habits
that will help them grow strong but not grow fat is to guide
their choice of high-calorie foods to those that contain large
amounts of protein and other nutrients as well as calories. For
example as snacks, drinks with a milk base are better than cola
drinks, peanut butter sandwiches better than potato chips, cheeseburgers better than candy bars.

Avoid Emotional Upset in Fat Teen-agers

It is easy to upset a teen-ager emotionally. The instability of
the quantity of hormones during and around puberty keeps the
adolescent in a state of touchiness. Girls are usually more emotional than boys at this age, and when upset, a child does not
digest or absorb food well. Therefore, even though a teen-ager
is overweight, it is unwise to berate him or her for "stuffing himself." Keep him on an even emotional keel as much as possible
by not nagging, or cutting down too much on amount of snacks
or other food he eats. But try to lead him intelligently into eating
quantities of food with the protein, calcium and other nutrients
he needs, instead of mountains of food with empty calories and
little more.

Dr. Sebrell states that breakfast of fruit or fruit juice, cereal with
milk, two slices of bread and a glass of milk provides a nutritious
teen-age breakfast, especially when an egg or a slice of ham is

added. No matter how overweight a teen-ager is, he must eat a balanced breakfast that amounts to from one-third to one-fourth of his total daily food. Sebrell says the importance of a good breakfast for growing boys and girls cannot be overstressed. The tendency to skip breakfast by fat teens is dangerous to their health and is not the way to help them lose weight. Even though a child is fat, he must eat some food from each of these groups every day. Don't, for example, cut out potatoes, or bread, or even pie or cake, which he loves. But cut down on them; instead of four meat sandwiches for school lunch, give him three. Limit him to one instead of two potatoes, one piece of his favorite cake or pie, one bottle of soft drink a day instead of his usual two or three. Your purpose is to retard the growth of fat but at the same time not to retard the growth of bone and muscle, or to upset him emotionally.

Encourage Teen-agers to Use Bathroom Scales

Once a fat adolescent decides for himself, rather than under pressure from parents or relatives, that he really does want to look better, be more popular and feel stronger by losing ugly excess pounds, give him a bathroom scale. It is an important tool in teen-age weight control. How much he should weigh can be determined by weight and height and age tables. How much does he weigh? Encourage him to ask the bathroom scales before breakfast. Let him repeat his asking the scales regularly and at the same time of the day while he is trying to cut down his fat. Young people have to see results in order to be encouraged to continue losing weight.

Getting the teen-ager down to his normal weight according to age and height is only the beginning. The long-term purpose is to teach him that most blessed of habits in our overabundant era, namely, the habit of not getting fat. When an adolescent acquires that habit and enjoys it, he will, in all likelihood, avoid obesity as an adult.

CHAPTER 15

Group
Meals Help
Fat Teen-ager

THE ENVIRONMENT of a child often determines whether or not he will develop into an overweight adult. If he grows up in a family with good eating habits, the chances of his avoiding obesity, that most prevalent form of malnutrition and the most difficult to cure, are in his favor.

That is why the psychological, practical and example value of family meals for overweight young children and adolescents is stressed by child psychologists and diet therapists equally. But the family meals must be nutritionally balanced, enjoyable, and not in caloric excess of the energy needs of the most active and growing members of the family. Enjoyment of food plus nutrition, rather than overindulgence, should be the purpose of the family menus.

When a child grows up in the daily environment of nutritional sanity, good eating habits can become a form of enjoyment rather than a resented discipline. Under these favorable circumstances, a fat child ultimately can learn by imitation the habit of not staying fat. He will do this without loss of emotional stability through deep-seated resentment against parental threats, mockery and psychologically upsetting deprivation.

All Overweight Members of Family Can Profit by Family Meals

The overweight child is not the only member of the family to profit by family meals. Overweight fathers as well as mothers can profit. With very few exceptions, these meals offer the overweight adult also the best opportunity for a long-term weight-reduction program.

In a family where individual members are on various weight-reducing or weight-control diets, the person responsible for feeding the family can plan menus with malice toward none and compassion for all. The basic menus, nutritionally balanced, are for the growing children and non-dieting members. But from the basic menu the dieters, according to the number of calories they are allowed, can enjoy enough of the family meal to feel a sense of "belonging" rather than as one set apart. Of course, it may cost the dieter a little will power to pass up the second piece of pie. But he knows it would cost him a lot more to pay doctors to free him from the likely consequences of obesity.

The family meal is so important to the maintenance of long-term weight-reducing programs, to the re-education of the appetite, without which no diet can have permanent value, and to the training of overweight children in sound eating habits, that experienced diet therapists now encourage it. They regard it as one of the most practical and normal forms of group therapy.

The seven-day family menus that follow, with modifications at 1,200, 1,500 and 1,800 calories a day are based on familiar, grocery store foods at moderate cost in interesting variety. They were prepared by Elizabeth K. Caso, M.S., instructor in nutrition at the Harvard University School of Public Health, and chairman, Diet Therapy Section of The American Dietetic Association, 1956-1959.

Week's Menus for the Family with a Dieter

SUNDAY

For the Family   *1,800 Calories*

BREAKFAST

Grapefruit sections (fresh or canned unsweetened)	Grapefruit sections (fresh or canned unsweetened)
Grilled Canadian bacon	Canadian bacon, lean, 2 slices
Pancakes, syrup, butter	Pancakes, 2 medium
	Butter, 1 teaspoon
	Syrup, 2 teaspoons
Coffee	Coffee, black *or* with part of day's portion of milk

DINNER

Roast sirloin of beef, gravy	Roast sirloin of beef, 3 ounces, no gravy
Pan-baked potatoes	Baked potato, plain, 1 small
Butter	Butter, 3 teaspoons for potato, vegetable, roll
Fresh, canned or frozen asparagus, butter	Fresh, canned or frozen asparagus, 8 to 10 stalks
Stuffed celery, carrot curls	Plain celery, carrot curls
Hot rolls, butter	Roll, plain, 1 small
Vanilla ice cream, butterscotch sauce, chopped almonds	Vanilla ice cream, 1 cup with chopped almonds (extra treat)
Coffee, milk	Coffee

EVENING SNACK

Tomato bouillon, crackers	Tomato bouillon, 4 crackers
Assorted sandwiches (make your own)	Sandwich
	Rye bread, 2 slices
	Cold tongue, 3 thin slices
	lettuce, mustard, horseradish
Chocolate layer cake	Pear, fresh, 1 medium
	Gruyère cheese, 1 wedge
Milk	Milk, 1 glass (8 ounces)

SUNDAY

1,500 Calories　　　　　　　　　*1,200 Calories*

BREAKFAST

Grapefruit sections (fresh or
　canned unsweetened)
Canadian bacon, lean, 1 slice
Toast, 1 slice
Butter, 1 teaspoon
Coffee, black *or* with part of
　day's portion of milk

Grapefruit sections (fresh or
　canned unsweetened)
Canadian bacon, lean, 1 slice
Toast, 1 slice, no butter

Coffee, black *or* with part of
　day's portion of milk

DINNER

Roast sirloin of beef, 3 ounces,
　no gravy
Baked potato, plain, 1 small
Fresh, canned or frozen aspara-
　gus, 8 to 10 stalks
Butter, 2 teaspoons for potato,
　vegetable
Plain celery, carrot curls
Roll, plain, 1 small, no butter
Vanilla ice cream, ½ cup with
　chopped almonds (extra
　treat)
Coffee

Roast sirloin of beef, 3 ounces,
　no gravy

Fresh, canned or frozen aspara-
　gus, 8 to 10 stalks, no butter

Plain celery, carrot curls
Roll, plain, 1 small, no butter
Vanilla ice cream, ½ cup with
　chopped almonds (extra
　treat)
Coffee

EVENING SNACK

Tomato bouillon, 4 crackers
Sandwich
　Rye bread, 2 slices
　Cold tongue, 3 thin slices
　lettuce, mustard, horseradish
Pear, fresh, 1 medium
Gruyère cheese, 1 wedge
Milk, 1 glass (8 ounces)

Tomato bouillon, fat-free
Sandwich
　Rye bread, 1 slice
　Cold tongue, 3 thin slices
　lettuce, mustard, horseradish
Pear, fresh, 1 medium

Milk, 1 glass (8 ounces)

MONDAY

For the Family   *1,800 Calories*

BREAKFAST

Melon *or* Grapefruit	Melon *or* Grapefruit
Oatmeal with chopped dates, cream, sugar	Oatmeal, plain, ½ cup, no sugar, part of milk allowed for day
	Egg, soft-boiled, 1 teaspoon butter
Toast, butter	Toast, 1 slice, 1 teaspoon butter
Coffee	Coffee
Milk	

LUNCH

Roast beef hash, catsup	Cold roast beef, 2 small slices (2 ounces)
	Potato salad
	1 small potato, chopped onion, parsley, vinegar, lettuce
Pickles, olives, celery, radishes	Celery, radishes
Bread, butter	
Fruit gelatin, whipped cream	Peaches, canned, unsweetened, 2 halves
	Cookie, plain, 1 medium
Milk	Milk, 1 glass (8 ounces)

DINNER

Barbecued spareribs	Broiled pork tenderloin, 4 ounces
	Barbecue sauce, 3 teaspoons
Corn niblets	Corn niblets, ½ cup, 1 teaspoon butter
Tomato and chicory salad, Roquefort dressing	Tomato and chicory salad, 2 teaspoons French dressing
Garlic bread	Garlic bread, 1 slice
Dutch apple cake, vanilla sauce	Apple, fresh, 1 small
Coffee	Coffee
Milk	

MONDAY

1,500 Calories   *1,200 Calories*

BREAKFAST

Melon *or* Grapefruit   Melon *or* Grapefruit
Egg, soft-boiled, 1 teaspoon but-   Egg, soft-boiled
  ter
Oatmeal, plain, ½ cup, no sugar,   Oatmeal, plain, ½ cup, no sugar,
  part of milk allowed for day   part of milk allowed for day
Coffee   Coffee

LUNCH

Cold roast beef, 2 small slices   Cold roast beef, 1 small slice (1
  (2 ounces)   ounce)
Potato salad   Potato salad
  1 small potato, chopped   1 small potato, chopped on-
  onion, parsley, vinegar, let-   ion, parsley, vinegar, lettuce
  tuce
Celery, radishes   Celery, radishes
Peaches, canned, unsweetened,   Peaches, canned unsweetened,
  2 halves   2 halves
Cookie, plain, 1 medium
Milk, 1 glass (8 ounces)   Milk, 1 glass (8 ounces)

DINNER

Broiled pork tenderloin, lean, 3   Broiled pork tenderloin, lean, 3
  ounces   ounces
Barbecue sauce, 3 teaspoons   Barbecue sauce 2 teaspoons
Corn niblets, ½ cup, 1 teaspoon   Corn niblets, ½ cup, no butter
  butter
Tomato and chicory salad, herb   Tomato and chicory salad, herb
  dressing (no oil)   dressing (no oil)
Garlic bread, 1 slice   Garlic bread, ½ slice
Apple, fresh, 1 small   Apple, fresh, 1 small
Coffee   Coffee

TUESDAY

For the Family   *1,800 Calories*

BREAKFAST

Chilled orange juice	Chilled orange juice, ½ cup
Poached eggs on toasted corn bread	Poached egg, 1
	Corn bread, 2 pieces (1½-inch cube)
Butter	Butter, 2 teaspoons
Coffee	Coffee
Milk	

LUNCH

Grilled cheese sandwiches	Grilled cheese sandwich
	bread, 2 slices
	fat, 1 teaspoon
	cheese, 2 ounces
Cole slaw, sour cream dressing	Cole slaw, 1 tablespoon sour cream dressing
Chocolate pudding, cream	Pineapple, fresh or canned unsweetened, ½ cup
Coconut cookies	
Milk	Milk, 1 glass (8 ounces)

DINNER

Baked meat loaf, tomato sauce	Broiled hamburger patty, 4 ounces
String beans with mushrooms	String beans, mushrooms, no butter
French fried potatoes	Carrots with chopped parsley
Caraway seed rolls	Roll, 1 small
Butter	Butter, 1 teaspoon
Lemon chiffon pie	Lemon sherbet, 1 cup
Coffee	Coffee
Milk	

TUESDAY

1,500 Calories   *1,200 Calories*

BREAKFAST

Chilled orange juice, ½ cup   Chilled orange juice, ½ cup
Poached egg, 1   Poached egg, 1
Corn bread, 1 piece (1½-inch   Corn bread, 1 piece (1½-inch
  cube)   cube)
Butter, 1 teaspoon   No butter
Coffee   Coffee

LUNCH

Grilled cheese sandwich   Open-faced broiled cheese sand-
  bread, 2 slices   wich
  fat, 1 teaspoon   bread, 1 slice
  cheese, 2 ounces   tomato, 1 slice
                                       cheese, 1 ounce
Cole slaw, 1 tablespoon sour   Cole slaw, Zero salad dressing
  cream dressing   (see recipe, pp. 140-141)
Pineapple, fresh or canned un-   Pineapple, fresh or canned, unsweetened, ½ cup   sweetened, ½ cup
Milk, 1 glass (8 ounces)   Milk, 1 glass (8 ounces)

DINNER

Broiled hamburger patty, 3   Broiled hamburger patty, 3
  ounces   ounces
String beans, mushrooms, no   String beans, mushrooms, no
  butter   butter
Carrots with chopped parsley   Carrots with chopped parsley
Roll, 1 small   Roll, 1 small
Butter, 1 teaspoon   Butter, 1 teaspoon
Lemon sherbet, ½ cup   Lemon gelatin (see recipe, p.
                                      137)

Coffee   Coffee

WEDNESDAY

For the Family   *1,800 Calories*

BREAKFAST

Sliced banana   Sliced banana, ½, small
Dry cereal, sugar, cream   Dry cereal, ¾ cup, no sugar, part
                                      of milk allowed for day
Bran raisin muffins, butter   Plain bran muffin, 1 small
                                   Butter, 1 teaspoon
Coffee   Coffee
Milk

LUNCH

Avocado half, stuffed with crab-   Tomato stuffed with crabmeat
  meat   ¾ cup crabmeat
                                      celery
                                      2 teaspoons of mayonnaise
French rolls, butter   French roll, 1 small, no butter
Hot gingerbread, whipped cream   Gingerbread, 1 small square (2
                                      x 2 x 1½-inches)
Milk   Milk, 1 glass (8 ounces)

DINNER

Broiled lamb chops   Broiled lamb chop, lean, 4
                                      ounces (2 rib or 1 large kid-
                                      ney chop)
Mint jelly
Baked squash   Baked squash
                                   Butter, 1 teaspoon
Mashed potatoes   Mashed potato, prepared with
                                      ½ cup milk, no butter
Bread, butter   Bread, 1 slice
                                   Butter, 1 teaspoon
Apricot upside-down cake   Apricots, 4 halves, unsweetened
                                      (fresh, canned or dried)
Coffee   Coffee
Milk

WEDNESDAY

1,500 Calories   *1,200 Calories*

BREAKFAST

Sliced banana, ½ small
Dry cereal, ¾ cup, no sugar, part
    of milk allowed for day
Coffee

Sliced banana, ½ small
Dry cereal, ¾ cup, no sugar,
    part of milk allowed for day
Coffee

LUNCH

Tomato, stuffed with crabmeat
    ¾ cup crabmeat
    celery
    2 teaspoons of mayonnaise
French roll, 1 small, no butter
Plums, 2 medium (fresh or
    canned unsweetened)
        or
Tangerine, 1
Milk, 1 glass (8 ounces)

Tomato stuffed with crabmeat
    ½ cup crabmeat
    celery
    lemon juice
French roll, 1 small, no butter
Plums, 2 medium (fresh or
    canned unsweetened)
        or
Tangerine, 1
Milk, 1 glass (8 ounces)

DINNER

Broiled lamb chop, lean, 3
    ounces (2 rib or 1 large kid-
    ney chop)
Baked squash
Butter, 1 teaspoon
Mashed potato, prepared with
    ½ cup milk, no butter
Bread, 1 slice
Butter, 1 teaspoon
Apricots, 4 halves unsweetened,
    (fresh, canned or dried)
Coffee

Broiled lamb chop, lean, 3
    ounces (2 rib or 1 large kid-
    ney chop)
Baked squash
Butter, 1 teaspoon
Mashed potato, prepared with ½
    cup milk, no butter

Apricots, 4 halves, unsweetened
    (fresh, canned or dried)
Coffee

THURSDAY

For the Family   *1,800 Calories*

BREAKFAST

Chilled orange juice   Chilled orange juice, ½ cup
Scrambled eggs   Scrambled eggs (no fat) 1 por-
                                      tion
Broiled sausages   Broiled sausage, 1
Toast   Toast, 2 slices
Butter   Butter, 1 teaspoon
Coffee   Coffee
Milk

LUNCH

Cream of tomato soup   Cream of tomato soup (with
                                      milk)
Croutons   Croutons, 8 to 10
Cottage cheese and chopped   Cottage cheese and chopped
  pepper salad, French dressing   pepper salad, ½ cup
                                    French dressing, 2 teaspoons
Whole-wheat roll, butter   Whole-wheat roll, 1 small, no
                                      butter
Apple turnover   Apple, fresh, 1 small, *or*
                                      Cinnamon applesauce, un-
                                      sweetened, ½ cup
Milk   Milk, 1 glass (6 ounces)

DINNER

Cranberry juice cocktail
Baked chicken, Parmesan   Broiled chicken, paprika, ½, no
                                      fat
Parsley potatoes   Parsley potato, 1 small
Green peas and diced carrots   Green peas, ½ cup
                                    Butter, 2 teaspoons for vegetable
                                      and potato
Corn muffins, butter
                                    Celery, carrot sticks, scallions
Grapenut pudding, cream   Grapenut pudding, ½ cup with
                                      milk
Coffee   Coffee
Milk

THURSDAY

1,500 Calories   *1,200 Calories*

BREAKFAST

Chilled orange juice, ½ cup

Scrambled egg (no fat), 1 portion

Toast, 1 slice

Butter, 1 teaspoon

Coffee

Chilled orange juice, ½ cup

Scrambled egg (no fat), 1 portion

Toast, 1 slice, no butter

Coffee

LUNCH

Cream of tomato soup (with
milk)

Croutons, 8 to 10

Cottage cheese and chopped
pepper salad, ½ cup

French dressing, 2 teaspoons

Whole-wheat roll, 1 small, no
butter

Apple, fresh, 1 small *or*
Cinnamon applesauce, un-
sweetened, ½ cup

Milk, 1 glass (6 ounces)

Tomato bouillon, fat-free

Cottage cheese and chopped
pepper salad, ½ cup

Zero salad dressing

Whole-wheat roll, 1 small, no
butter

Apple, fresh, 1 small *or*
Cinnamon applesauce, un-
sweetened, ½ cup

Milk, 1 glass (8 ounces)

DINNER

Broiled chicken, paprika, ½, no
fat

Parsley potato, 1 small

Green peas, ½ cup

Butter, 2 teaspoons for vegetable
and potato

Celery, carrot sticks, scallions

Grapes, 12

Coffee

Broiled chicken, paprika, ¼, no
fat

Parsley potato, 1 small

Green peas, ½ cup

Butter, 1 teaspoon for vegetables
and potato

Celery, carrot sticks, scallions

Grapes, 12

Coffee

FRIDAY

For the Family   *1,800 Calories*

BREAKFAST

Grapefruit half or ½ cup canned
   sections unsweetened
French toast, syrup, butter

Broiled bacon
Blueberry muffins, butter
Coffee
Milk

Grapefruit half or ½ cup canned
   sections unsweetened
French toast, 2 slices (cooked
   in 2 teaspoons of fat)
Syrup, 3 teaspoons

Coffee

LUNCH

Tuna fish, noodle casserole

Mixed green salad
Chiffonade dressing
Bread, butter
Strawberries, cream *or* Fresh
   orange sections
Oatmeal cookies
Milk

Tuna fish, noodle casserole
   Tuna fish, ½ cup
   Cooked noodles, 1 cup
   Onion flakes
   Seasoning
   Butter, 1 teaspoon
Mixed green salad
Zero dressing

Strawberries, fresh, 1 cup with
   milk, *or* Fresh orange sections

Milk, 1 glass (6 ounces)

DINNER

Broiled halibut steak, lemon
   butter
Potato croquettes
Harvard beets
Jellied cabbage salad
Mayonnaise
Poppyseed rolls
Butter
Maple walnut layer cake
Coffee
Milk

Broiled halibut steak, 4 ounces,
   wedge lemon
Baked potato, 1 small
Pickled beets (no sugar)
Jellied cabbage salad
Mayonnaise, 1 teaspoon
Poppyseed roll, 1 small
Butter, 1 teaspoon
Fresh fruit cup, ½ cup
Coffee

FRIDAY

1,500 Calories   *1,200 Calories*

BREAKFAST

Grapefruit half or ½ cup canned   Grapefruit half or ½ cup canned
   sections unsweetened   sections unsweetened
Egg, soft-boiled, 1   Egg, soft-boiled, 1
Muffin, plain, 1 (2-inch diam-   Muffin, plain, 1 (2-inch diam-
   eter)   eter)
Butter, 1 teaspoon   No butter
Coffee   Coffee

LUNCH

Tuna fish, noodle casserole   Tuna fish, noodle casserole
   Tuna fish, ½ cup   Tuna fish, ¼ cup
   Cooked noodles, 1 cup   Cooked noodles, ½ cup
   Onion flakes   Onion flakes
   Seasoning   Seasoning
   Butter, 1 teaspoon   No butter
Mixed green salad   Mixed green salad
Zero dressing   Zero dressing
Strawberries, fresh, 1 cup with   Strawberries, fresh, 1 cup with
   milk, *or* Fresh orange sections   milk, *or* Fresh orange sections
Milk, 1 glass (6 ounces)   Milk, 1 glass (6 ounces)

DINNER

Broiled halibut steak, 3 ounces,   Broiled halibut steak, 3 ounces,
   wedge lemon   wedge lemon
Baked potato, 1 small
Pickled beets (no sugar)   Pickled beets (no sugar)
Jellied cabbage salad   Jellied cabbage salad
Mayonnaise, 1 teaspoon   No dressing
Poppyseed roll, 1 small   Poppyseed roll, 1 small
Butter, 1 teaspoon   Butter, 1 teaspoon
Fresh fruit cup, ½ cup   Fresh fruit cup, ½ cup
Coffee   Coffee

SATURDAY

For the Family   *1,800 Calories*

BREAKFAST

Chilled orange juice   Chilled orange juice, ½ cup
Dry cereal, sugar, cream   Dry cereal, ¾ cup, no sugar, part
                                    of day's portion of milk
Sweet rolls   Toast, 1 slice
Butter   Butter, 1 teaspoon
Coffee   Coffee
Milk

LUNCH

Cheeseburgers on buns   Cheeseburger
                                    Hamburger, 2 ounces
                                    Roll, 1
                                    Cooking fat, 1 teaspoon
                                    Cheese, 1 ounce
Pickle relish   Relish, 1 teaspoon
Sliced tomatoes and cucumbers   Sliced tomatoes and cucumbers
French dressing   French dressing, 1 teaspoon
Chocolate ice cream sundae   Pear, fresh, 1 medium
Milk   Milk, 1 glass (6 ounces)

DINNER

Baked ham steak with sliced   Baked ham steak, 4 ounces
    pineapple
Scalloped potatoes   Broccoli
Broccoli   Hollandaise sauce, 1 teaspoon
Hollandaise sauce   Summer squash *or* Zucchini, 1
                                    cup
Rye bread   Rye bread, 1 slice
Butter   Butter, 1 teaspoon for vegetables
                                    and bread
Coconut cream pudding   Coconut cream pudding, ½ cup
                                    with milk
Coffee   Coffee
Milk

SATURDAY

1,500 Calories   *1,200 Calories*

BREAKFAST

Chilled orange juice, ½ cup   Chilled orange juice, ½ cup
Dry cereal, ¾ cup, no sugar,   Dry cereal, ¾ cup, no sugar,
   part of day's portion of milk   part of day's portion of milk
Coffee   Coffee

LUNCH

Cheeseburger   Cheeseburger
   Hamburger, 2 ounces   Hamburger, 1 ounce
   Roll, 1   Roll, ½
   Cooking fat, 1 teaspoon
   Cheese, 1 ounce   Cheese, 1 ounce
Relish, 1 teaspoon   Relish, 1 teaspoon
Sliced tomatoes and cucumbers   Sliced tomatoes and cucumbers
French dressing, 1 teaspoon   Zero dressing
Pear, fresh, 1 medium   Pear, fresh, 1 medium
Milk, 1 glass (6 ounces)   Milk, 1 glass (6 ounces)

DINNER

Baked ham steak, lean, 3 ounces   Baked ham steak, lean, 3 ounces
Broccoli   Broccoli
Hollandaise sauce, 1 teaspoon   Hollandaise sauce, 1 teaspoon
Summer squash *or* Zucchini, 1   Summer squash *or* Zucchini, 1
   cup   cup
Butter, 1 teaspoon for vegetables   Butter, 1 teaspoon for vegetables
                                        and bread
                                     Rye bread, 1 slice
Coconut cream pudding, ½ cup   Pineapple, canned, unsweet-
   with milk   ened, 1 slice
Coffee   Coffee

Seasonings

Seasoning of unbuttered vegetables and other foods is important to increase their palatability. The following seasonings may be used freely, if desired:

Chopped parsley	Mint
Garlic	Onion
Celery	Nutmeg
Mustard	Cinnamon
Pepper and other spices	Saccharin
Lemon	Vinegar

Special Notes

On 1,200-calorie diet, skim milk may be used in place of whole milk, if desired. Then 4 teaspoons of butter may be added for the day.

A 3-ounce portion of cooked meat or fish is equal to approximately 4 ounces, or ¼ pound raw.

Coffee on all calorie-restricted diets may be taken black or part of day's portion of milk may be used. One pint of milk is included daily in each diet plan.

A mid-afternoon or evening snack is planned for each diet consisting of part of the total amount of milk allowed for the day (1 pint), plus 4 to 6 small thin crackers. Plain tea, tomato juice, clear bouillon may also be used as "fill-ins."

CHAPTER 16

Men Diet Too

A FACT OFTEN overlooked by dieters is that men and women live in the world together. Fashion considerations and the deep-seated yearning of most women for the figure of a cover girl, have slanted much popular writing on weight reduction toward the feminine side of the dinner table.

Nevertheless, the basic principles of weight control apply equally to men and women. Any difference between reduction diets for men and women is only one of quantity, not of kind. Reduction in calories, re-education in eating habits, emotional stability and moderate regular exercise are factors over and above considerations of sex. That, however, is not to say that scientific reducing diets as a rule fail to increase the dieter's attractiveness —a matter of admitted interest to men and women alike.

A diet routine specially planned to trim down the moderately overweight man of the sedentary type, that is business executive, teacher, etc.—in general, the so-called white-collar overweight— is geared to his environment and cultural pattern, rather than to any physiological difference between him and his feminine counterpart except in calorie needs. In general, a man in this group uses around 2,400 calories a day; a woman, only 2,000.

A Man Should Estimate His Calorie Requirements

That is only a general estimate. For an estimate based on his individual needs, a man should first figure his desirable weight according to height and build (see page 23), then allow 16 calories for each pound of his weight. This will be the approximate number of calories needed to maintain his desirable weight.

For example, according to the tables, a man 5 feet 8 inches tall, of medium frame, should weigh about 145 to 156 pounds. Taking the figure 156 and multiplying it by 16, the answer is 2,496 calories, or the number needed to maintain him at his desirable weight. Admittedly, that figure is on the generous side. He probably could do well with less, provided his meals are nutritionally balanced and embrace a variety of foods.

However, a menu plan that totals approximately 2,200 calories a day can help a man lose weight slowly and with a reasonable amount of happiness. He has probably been eating much more than that and added extra pounds so gradually they were not noticed, except by his tailor.

Dr. Stare, apostle of "cut down, don't cut out," for overweight people, tested the following seven-day 2,200-calorie menu plan on a group of desk-worker men who were moderately overweight. His purpose was to induce them to learn to eat nutritionally sound meals with fewer, but not drastically fewer, calories. Therefore, the actual menus, prepared by his co-workers in the Department of Nutrition at Harvard University, are based on the kinds and variety of foods most men like and are used to eating.

Although the calorie allowances are a little low for most men, they are a little high for most women. But if a man and woman living together both use this basic pattern in the interests of practical household management while each is trying to reduce, it is easy enough to eliminate from the basic menus food to the value of 500 or more calories to bring it down to 1,700 or less for one person without losing the variety and balance.

American Wives Overstuff Their Men

Men customarily complain—and justly in many cases—that it is almost impossible to diet at home because their wives insist on serving calorie-rich foods. American wives have so long been told that the way to a man's heart is through his stomach, it is difficult for eager and devoted wives not to serve fancy meals. However, in the interest of both winning their hearts and keeping those hearts beating longer, modern women are listening more and more to medical and dietetic counselors, and learning to plan calorically lower meals that will give pleasure, nutrition, and longer life expectancy.

The Stare diet lends itself perfectly to the "Tea for Two" theme, providing good food, sound nutrition, and fewer calories for both husband and wife. Certainly, when both go on a weight-reduction program together, at the same table, the chances for emotional balance and long-term success are materially increased. Particularly, if they like each other.

Seven-Day 2,200 Calorie Diet

FIRST DAY

BREAKFAST

Orange juice, 4 ounces
Cereal, 1 serving
Milk, 1 cup
Toast, 1 slice
Jelly, 1 tablespoon
Coffee *or* Tea

LUNCH OR SUPPER

Bouillon
Cold roast beef, 2 ounces, sandwich with mustard
Sliced tomato
Strawberry shortcake (biscuit and sweetened berries)
Milk, 1 cup
Coffee *or* Tea

DINNER

Tomato juice cocktail
Broiled halibut, 4 ounces
Butter, 1 pat for cooking
Parsley potato
Butter, 1 pat
French-style green beans, 1 serving
Roll, 1
Jelly, 1 tablespoon
Grapefruit-orange salad
Jello
Coffee *or* Tea

BETWEEN-MEALS SNACKS
(Choice of one)

Soft drink, 1
Fruit juice, 4 ounces average
Milk, 1 cup
Graham crackers, 4
or
Plain cookies, 2

SECOND DAY

BREAKFAST

Prunes, ½ cup
Poached egg
Toast, 2 slices
Butter, 1 pat
Jelly, 1 tablespoon
Coffee *or* Tea

LUNCH OR SUPPER

Shrimp salad
  Shrimp, ½ cup
  Boiled dressing, 3 tablespoons
  Lettuce
  Seasoning
Grape juice cocktail, 4 ounces
Melba toast, 2 slices
Jam, 1 tablespoon
Pineapple sherbet (water)
Coffee *or* Tea
Milk, 1 cup

DINNER

Roast beef, 4 ounces
Boiled potato, 1 medium
Peas, 1 serving
Roll, 1
Butter, 1 pat
Tomato aspic salad
Angel cake, 1 serving
Frozen apricots, 1 serving
Coffee *or* Tea

BETWEEN-MEALS SNACKS
(Choice of one)

Soft drink, 1
Fruit juice, 4 ounces average
Milk, 1 cup
Graham crackers, 4
        or
Plain cookies, 2

THIRD DAY

BREAKFAST

Tangerine juice, 4 ounces
Cereal, 1 serving
Blueberry muffin, 1
Jam, 1 tablespoon
Milk, 1 cup
Coffee *or* Tea

LUNCH OR SUPPER

Fruit salad plate: pear, apple,
  cottage cheese, orange, banana

DINNER

Consommé, 1 serving
Saltines, 3
Lean roast leg of lamb, 3 slices
  (3 x 2¾ x ⅛-inches)
Glazed curried peach, ½
Brussels sprouts, 1 serving
Parsley buttered potato, 1 serv-
  ing
Cloverleaf rolls, 2
Butter, 1 pat
Lime ice, ½ cup

Butter, 1 pat
Toast, 2 slices
Plum jam, 2 tablespoons
Coffee *or* Tea

Jam, 1 tablespoon
Coffee *or* Tea

BETWEEN-MEALS SNACKS
(Choice of one)

Soft drink, 1
Fruit juice, 4 ounces average
Milk, 1 cup
Graham crackers, 4
or
Plain cookies, 2

FOURTH DAY

BREAKFAST

Orange juice, ½ cup
Cereal, 1 cup
Milk, 1 cup
Sugar, 1 teaspoon
Egg
Toast, 1 slice
Jam, 1 tablespoon
Coffee *or* Tea

LUNCH OR SUPPER

French onion soup with 4 saltines
Liverwurst on rye
Tomato, 1 medium, stuffed with Cottage cheese, ¼ cup, on Lettuce cup
Angel cake, 1 piece
Coffee *or* Tea

DINNER

Shrimp cocktail, 5 shrimp
Sauce, 4 tablespoons
Broiled chicken, ¼ medium broiler
Rice, ¾ cup with 1 pat butter
French-style green beans, ½ cup seasoned with thyme, green onion
Endive, lettuce, grapefruit salad with oil and vinegar dressing
Oil, 1½ teaspoons
Rolls, 2 small
Guava jelly, 2 tablespoons
Fruit
Coffee *or* Tea

BETWEEN-MEALS SNACKS
(Choice of one)

Soft drink, 1
Fruit juice, 4 ounces average
Milk, 1 cup
Graham crackers, 4
or
Plain cookies, 2

FIFTH DAY

BREAKFAST

Medium grapefruit, ½
Soft-cooked egg, 1
Whole-wheat toast, 2 slices
Strawberry jam, 1 tablespoon
Coffee *or* Tea

LUNCH OR SUPPER

Breast of chicken, ¼ large
  chicken
  Oil, 2 teaspoons for cooking
  Mushroom caps on toast
  triangles
Celery hearts and radishes
Broccoli with lemon
Sponge cake
Milk, 1 cup
Coffee *or* Tea

DINNER

Tomato bouillon
Saltines, 2
Roast lamb, 4 ounces
Mint jelly, 1 tablespoon
Steamed rice, ½ cup
Baked acorn squash, ½
Tossed salad with lemon juice
Butter, 1 pat
Parkerhouse roll, 1 small
Meringue filled with frozen
  cherries
Coffee *or* Tea

BETWEEN-MEALS SNACKS
(Choice of one)

Soft drink, 1
Fruit juice, 4 ounces average
Milk, 1 cup
Graham crackers, 4
or
Plain cookies, 2

SIXTH DAY

BREAKFAST

Sliced orange
Cereal, 1 cup
Milk, 1 cup
Sugar, 1 teaspoon
Toast, 1 slice
Strawberry jam, 1 tablespoon
Coffee *or* Tea

LUNCH OR SUPPER

Roast veal, 3 ounces

DINNER

Lean baked pork loin, 4 ounces,
  seasoned with mustard,
  Worcestershire sauce
Baked potato, 1 medium with
  chives and 1 tablespoon sour
  cream
Broccoli, ½ cup
Lettuce salad with vinegar
Small roll, 1
Marmalade, 1 tablespoon

Spaghetti, ½ cup
Tomato sauce, ¼ cup
Frozen peas, ½ cup
Italian bread, 1 slice
Jelly, 1 tablespoon
Milk, 1 cup
Frozen peaches, ½ cup
Coffee *or* Tea

SEVENTH DAY

BREAKFAST

Large grapefruit, ½
Poached egg
Toast, 2 slices
Jam, 2 tablespoons
Coffee *or* Tea

LUNCH OR SUPPER

Tomato juice cocktail, 4 ounces
Saltines, 2
Toasted turkey sandwich
Sweet pickles, 2 small
Radishes, 2
Celery hearts
Fruit
Milk, 1 cup
Coffee *or* Tea

Lemon chiffon pie, 1 serving
Coffee *or* Tea

BETWEEN-MEALS SNACKS
(Choice of one)

Soft drink, 1
Fruit juice, 4 ounces average
Milk, 1 cup
Graham crackers, 4
or
Plain cookies, 2

DINNER

Jellied consommé
Saltines, 4
Broiled halibut, 4 ounces with
  lemon wedge
Parsley buttered potato, 1
  medium with Butter, 1 pat
Asparagus, 1 serving
Rolls, 2 small
Honey, 2 tablespoons (*or* 2
  tablespoons jam *or* marma-
  lade)
Mixed green salad with
  Sour cream, 1 tablespoon
Melon balls (fresh or frozen),
  ⅔ cup
Coffee *or* Tea

BETWEEN-MEALS SNACKS
(Choice of one)

Soft drink, 1
Fruit juice, 4 ounces average
Milk, 1 cup
Graham crackers, 4
or
Plain cookies, 2

Notes

1. The fat content of these menus is lower than in most current American menus.
2. Extra fat, gravy or rich desserts will defeat the purpose of this diet.
3. A pat of butter means butter which is cut at 64 pats to a pound or 7 grams a pat, or approximately 1¼ teaspoons.
4. No gravy is used as it is almost impossible to estimate the fat. This means that pan gravy, or whatever comes off a steak or roast, as well as thickened gravy or sauces, are not included in the menus.
5. Meat is trimmed of all visible fat before being served. No frying is permitted but very small amounts of fat may be allowed to prevent sticking and dryness. Broth or bouillon may help prevent dryness.
6. With careful planning, a small amount of butter or fat can be used for seasoning, but generally not more than 3 pats of butter or other fat a day.
7. The use of generous amounts of non-fat milk and of fish, seafood, chicken, turkey or veal prepared with little or no fat is a good method for keeping a high protein intake and helping keep down the fat.
8. Vinegar, lemon, onion juice, spices and herbs may help season vegetables and meat.
9. If a bedtime snack is desired, it is suggested that those who are reducing or having trouble maintaining their weight, save their dessert for this snack.
10. Plain lettuce and tomato salad (without dressing) may be on the menu for any lunch or dinner.
11. One teaspoon of sugar and one teaspoon of whole milk may be added to each cup of coffee or tea as desired.

PART V

MISINFORMATION
AND
SUPERSTITION
CAN THWART
THE DIETER

CHAPTER 17

Effect of Fats on Heart Disease Unproven

CALORIES are the prima donnas of weight control. They get the spotlight in every discussion of overweight, whether it be a scientific discussion or merely an emotional jag caused by large draughts of current misinformation.

Eighty-five to ninety percent of the calories in our American diet generally come from carbohydrates and fat. Fat, however, is the most concentrated source of food energy, providing more than twice the number of calories derived from proteins or carbohydrates. Therefore, it is just good sense to cut down on fat as well as carbohydrates if you are overweight.

There is a great difference, however, between cutting down fat in the diet in order to cut down calories and the current hysteria about fat as a cause of heart disease and atherosclerosis.

Intensive dietary, medical and biochemical research have not yet proved conclusively that certain kinds of animal fats in the diet are the specific cause of arterial and heart disease. Premature conclusions, nevertheless, are often dramatically publicized. The result is widespread confusion in the public mind and even among practicing physicians.

The free-for-all debate on unsaturated (soft) and saturated (hard) fats, their influence on the amount of cholesterol in the blood stream, and the effects of even a slight increase of cholesterol on the arteries and heart is befuddling, sensational and frightening. Most of it results from incomplete evidence flamboyantly presented.

The majority of the leading research scientists are still unconvinced that moderate changes in blood cholesterol furnish a reliable index to the effect of different diets upon risks of heart attack. But they are learning rapidly what dietary factors regulate cholesterol concentration.

Contrary to the wave of fear about fat in our diet, these research scientists have not yet identified the key factors that cause heart attacks. The problem is very complex, they warn the dieting public. Therefore, indulging in fads, miracle diets and other extreme practices is hazardous and against scientific advice.

Both Saturated and Unsaturated Fats Belong in Balanced Diet

According to Dr. C. G. King, director of much of the intensive research in university and clinical laboratories on the relationship between cholesterol and heart disease, hardening of the arteries and cerebral "strokes," most scientists now recognize that both unsaturated and saturated fats have a respectable and valuable place in our diets.

"The two best guides for better health at present," he counsels, "are first to maintain a well-balanced and varied diet, and secondly, to control body weight by limiting the caloric intake to keep it in balance with physical work and exercise."

He does not deny that there are strong indications that when we understand more clearly how to control avoidable disturbances in fat metabolism in the human body, we will be better able to postpone and decrease heart disease and related conditions. He agrees further that linoleic acid in edible fats and oils is useful in maintaining balance in the diet. More factors in maintaining balance are other fatty acids such as those in the body fat of fish, mineral intake with emphasis on magnesium, and the physical mechanisms that regulate blood clotting and bile secretion.

Dr. King, executive director of the Nutrition Foundation, cautions the apprehensive dieter against uninformed decisions concerning the use of corn, cottonseed, soybean and peanut oil (unsaturated fats) as against margarines and hydrogenated vegetable and animal oils (saturated fats). There are indications, but not yet proof, that *overemphasis* on saturated fats may be one of many factors conducive to heart disease. But he states positively that research has proved that there are a number of variable factors that effect the disease. No one or two can be tagged as specific.

Many Factors Cause of Heart Disease

Among the unquestionable factors in the cause of heart disease (experimental and clinical) and related conditions, scientists list the following:

1. Genetic—The inherited physical tendency toward arterial and heart diseases.
2. High Blood Pressure.
3. Environment—Unfavorable sanitation, weather, clothing, bacterial infections, chemical exposure, smoking, emotional stress.
4. Overweight.
5. Nutrition—Inadequate amounts of protein or choline, excess calcium and deficient magnesium. In general, poorly balanced diets.
6. Tendency toward inadequate control of blood clotting. A large part of the problem.
7. Tendency toward poor liver functioning. Good quality protein is one of the best means to maintain healthy state of the liver.

Dr. King points out that though these factors are known to affect the arteries and heart adversely, no one can say in what combination they must work to produce unfavorable results. He stresses this fact also: most conservative researches and mature fundamental studies emphasize that we do not yet know of any one basic cause of heart disease.

For these reasons it is obvious that highly publicized campaigns against use of foods containing cholesterol are based only on fragmentary data and premature conclusions. The Nutrition Foundation alone is now supporting research on the human metabolism of fats at the Rockefeller Foundation, Johns Hopkins University, Columbia University, the University of Pennsylvania, the University of Chicago, Washington University, Harvard University, Tulane University, the University of California and the University of Colorado. It supports also studies bearing on arteriosclerosis at the Institute of Nutrition in Central America and Panama and study linked to this research at the University of Wisconsin. Elsewhere in the United States and Canada, similar intensive research is being financed on the relationship between fats and heart disease.

Advise against Major Change in Basic American Diet

Until definite proof that cholesterol from food in the blood stream can cause heart and arterial diseases has been discovered, most biochemists, medical researchers and nutritionists advise against any major change in the basic American diet.

For example, the Food and Nutrition Board of the National Research Council (the supreme court of the American diet) reports (1958), it is not yet possible to state definitely a reasonable allowance for fat in the diet or to indicate the characteristics of a fatty acid mixture most favorable for the support of health. A diet selected from a wide variety of foodstuffs, both vegetable and animal, is most likely to maintain good health.

Dr. Grace A. Goldsmith, professor of medicine at Tulane University, believes there is little doubt that atherosclerosis is the result of a combination of many factors, including heredity, sex, anatomy of the blood-vessel walls, and arterial blood pressure, in addition to diet and fat content of blood. She concludes, "The evidence at present does not convey any specific implications for drastic dietary changes, specifically in the quantity or type of fat in the diet of the general population on the premise that such changes will definitely lessen the incidence of coronary or cerebral artery disease."

Her advice, like that of the majority of other students of obesity is (1) to make some reduction in the amount of dietary fat, because fat is the most concentrated source of calories; (2) to consume a varied diet which furnishes good protein from animal as well as plant sources, and enough fat to fulfill potential needs of essential fatty acids and to meet but not exceed calorie requirements.

Stick to Common-Sense Weight-Reduction Program

These statements from highly accredited scientific sources should help banish panic caused by sensational and unsound attacks on certain types of fat foods. Until the results of the vast amount of research now being done on the role of fats in heart and arterial diseases, the overweight dieter should stick to his common-sense weight-reduction program, cutting down reasonably, but not totally, on fat for the very obvious reason that fat is supercharged with calories.

Although the prime purpose of this book is to help men, women and children lose unneeded and often dangerous excess pounds, and keep them lost for a lifetime, it does also offer help to those who live in dread of heart disease. First, it urges reduction in calories to bring weight down to desirable averages. Second, it urges constant maintenance of desirable weight, discouraging the "on again, off again" system of drastic dieting followed by over-indulgence and regaining of weight. Third, it urges regular moderate exercise every day, to burn up calories, to keep the body toned and to release stress. All three of these disciplines, according to current scientific findings, can contribute to the prevention of heart disease.

CHAPTER 18

Self-Deception
a Dietary Luxury

STICKING to a weight-reduction program is definitely possible, but usually difficult and often painful.

It is not something the left hand can do while the right hand is unrestrained with the knife and fork. It is a two-fisted job requiring will power, a basic understanding of nutrition, emotional stability and regular exercise.

That is a rather large order for most of us poor weak mortals in an era of tensions and overabundance. We want to get rid of our excess pounds. We know they are a health hazard and detract from our appearance. But the devil in the story is our appetite.

Curbing Your Appetite

How can we curb our appetite, our seemingly unmanageable desire for more food than we need? By will power fueled by a passionate determination to eat less and exercise more—the only sure-fire formula for weight reduction and control.

Let's face it. Will power is fine and dandy, but a little magic would be quicker. The belief in magical methods of losing weight seems to increase proportionately with excess pounds. Our basic American horse sense, our proverbial "show me" attitude, melts before the lure of so-called appetite depressors, drugs and gadgets "guaranteed" to banish appetite and pounds without the need of will power. According to the American Medical Association estimate, otherwise intelligent Americans spend $100,000,000 a year on fraudulent weight reducers.

Many more millions are spent annually on pills, wafers and

drugs which, though not fraudulent in the legal sense, have little or no permanent effect on the appetite.

Appetite Depressors, Drugs and Gadgets

They fall into three groups: so-called appetite depressors in the form of candies, pills and wafers which contain sugar and milk solids and some vitamins. The manufacturers claim that if these are taken before meals they will cause the blood sugar to rise and therefore depress the desire to eat a large meal. Objective research in laboratories has not found these claims to be true. A five-cent bag of ordinary lemon drops would do as well as a box of these expensive, dubious and flamboyantly advertised "dietary aids" to reducing.

There are also bulk producers which are supposed to lessen your appetite by absorbing water and then swelling, thereby filling up your stomach. Clinical research does not find the appetite depressing claims for these bulkers justified. Radishes, celery, green onions, cucumber and carrot sticks nibbled before dinner will provide as much bulk, supply more nutrition and cost far less.

There are drugs which depress appetite by acting on the centers of the nervous system. A doctor's prescription is necessary for most of them. So is medical supervision to watch for frequent toxic effects. Also, after a few weeks or months, the patient develops a tolerance for them and the drugs then lose their earlier effectiveness.

Therefore, unless a qualified physician advises and prescribes these drugs for you, take a walk and save money. Regular exercise and a nutritionally balanced diet are more effective and more permanent means to weight reduction.

Another form of self-deception popular with the overweight is the mechanical hobby horse. It can take three forms—a table that vibrates in a luxurious salon, a similar device that does the same at home, and an electrical gadget that stimulates the muscles. Of course, in each case, you are given a reducing diet to follow while using the hobby horse. The diet works quite well. The gadget may be fun as a form of psychotherapy that helps the dieter stick to his weight-reduction program. But no one has yet been able to prove conclusively that any of these gadgets by itself caused him or her to lose a pound.

Because weight reduction is both a human as well as a scientific problem, room must be allowed for the pleasures of self-deception. Therefore, if using some of the gadgets or some of the non-injurious pills, or even drugs (with your doctor's permission), makes losing pounds and keeping them lost seem easier by providing a psychological crutch, very little harm is likely to result. Provided, of course, you do not deceive yourself on the one basic fact—the only way to lose weight is to eat less and exercise more.

Artificial Sweeteners

The use of artificial sweeteners instead of sugar in reducing diets is not a form of self-deception. But under some conditions it can be.

Fruits and soft drinks that are artificially sweetened can have a place in the reducing diet under certain circumstances. But you may be lulled into false security by them. According to the Food and Nutrition Board of the National Research Council, a distinct place exists for them in cases where sugar must be eliminated, as in diabetes. But they are being used increasingly by many who hope to lose weight painlessly. The Board has no objection to this use, but warns that unless definite calorie control is followed at the same time, there will not be any benefit. There is bound to be disappointment unless the dieter curbs his appetite along with the consumption of these artificial sweeteners (saccharin and Sucaryl).

For example, just because you pour calorie-free soft drinks into your highball glass, it does not follow that the calories in the alcohol are in any way reduced. Nor that a slice of rich chocolate cake, sweetened with Sucaryl is calorie-free. The butter, chocolate, milk and eggs have just as many calories as they ever did. All that is missing is the amount of calories there would have been if sugar was used.

The Salt-Free Diet

Salt-free diets also can trick the dieter. Cutting down on salt, unless recommended because of the common type of high blood pressure, will not help you. There are no calories in salt. Nevertheless, a decrease in use of salt usually results in a loss of body weight, but only because less water will be retained in the body tissues. That has nothing to do with losing body fat. Eating fewer calories does.

PART VI

USE OF
EXCHANGE
LISTS
MORE
PRACTICAL
THAN
CALORIE
COUNTING

CHAPTER 19

A Fair Exchange
Is No Robbery

A FAIR EXCHANGE is no robbery. That goes as well for calories as it does for merchandise.

Instead of calorie counting, at best a frustrating form of self-torture, many students of the problems of long-term weight control suggest meal planning with exchange lists. It is far more practical, does not require constant referring to calorie charts, and makes it possible to stay within a calorie budget without nervous strain.

If, for example, you have 70 calories to spend on bread, cereals and other forms of carbohydrates in a meal, you can exchange these 70 calories for any of the foods in the Bread Exchange list, all of which contain 70 calories. So, what will it be? A slice of bread, a roll, a muffin, cereals, dry and cooked, a small white potato, one piece of sponge cake, etc. Anything you like, provided it is in that particular exchange list.

That, of course, is an oversimplified explanation of the use of exchange lists. The system divides most of the commonly used American foods into six exchange lists. Because the foods are so familiar to you and because they are grouped pretty much as you, yourself, would group them, you can memorize these six groups within a day or two. Once you have made these groups part of your normal thinking, you can easily plan meals that fit your personal tastes, stay within calorie limitations, and are nutritionally balanced.

Include Some Food from Each of Six Exchange Lists Every Day

The system is based on two principles. First, your daily calorie allowance must be distributed among the kinds of food needed for a nutritionally balanced diet. Your daily meal plan must include some food from each of the six lists—milk, vegetables, fruit, bread and cereals, meat, and fat.

Second, within each group of essential foods, there are listed foods of the same calorie content and same general food value. For example, in the meat group, the following items each contain 75 calories, 7 grams of protein and 5 grams of fat:

1. One ounce of medium fat beef, lamb, pork, liver, chicken, etc.
2. Cold cuts (4½ x ⅛-inch) 1 slice salami, minced ham, bologna, liverwurst or luncheon loaf.
3. One frankfurter (8 to 9 to a pound).
4. One egg.
5. Fish—1 ounce haddock, ¼ cup canned fish such as salmon, tuna, crab, lobster or small shrimp, clams, oysters or 3 medium sardines.
6. Cheese—1 ounce cheddar cheese or ¼ cup cottage cheese.
7. Two tablespoons peanut butter.

As most reducing diets include at least 225 calories from protein in the day's main meal, you would normally allow yourself 3 meat exchanges for dinner. Therefore, using the exchange list and selecting according to your personal preference, you could eat any of the following triple exchanges, each totaling 225 calories and each the equivalent of the other in protein and fat: a pork chop weighing ¼ pound; a 3-egg omelet; 2 lamb chops weighing ¼ pound; ¼ pound roast beef or roast chicken; or a cold plate consisting of 1 hard-cooked egg, an ounce slice of ham and ¼ cup cottage cheese. Or you could select 2 meat balls weighing ¼ pound, or the same weight in broiled liver or fish.

Vegetables Are in Two Exchange Lists

Vegetables are divided into two exchange lists. List A vegetables contain so little carbohydrate, protein and calories, you may eat as many as you like raw (except tomatoes and tomato juice) and cooked as much as one cup at a time. Among the List A vegetables are asparagus, broccoli, celery, cabbage, cauliflower, lettuce, mushrooms and watercress.

List B vegetables contain 35 calories plus 7 grams of carbohydrate and 2 grams of protein. Among them are onions, beets, green peas, pumpkin, turnips; also carrots and winter squash, which contain a lot of vitamin A.

In your diet menu for one meal, therefore, ½ cup of any of these List B vegetables can be exchanged for 1 full cup of cooked List A vegetables.

Fruit exchanges, containing 40 calories, include ½ cup applesauce, ½ small banana, 1 small orange, 2 dried prunes, ½ cup grapefruit or orange juice. Therefore, if your diet breakfast menu calls for 4 ounces of orange juice, and you prefer some other fruit, you can for example exchange it for ½ cup grapefruit juice, ⅔ cup blueberries, ½ banana, etc., without upsetting the calorie count or nutritional balance.

Some vegetables are listed under the bread exchanges, all containing 70 calories. For example, 1 slice of bread can be exchanged for 1 small boiled potato, ½ cup mashed potato or ¼ cup sweet potato or yam. Or 2 graham crackers can be exchanged in your menu for ½ cup cooked dried lima or navy beans, split peas or cowpeas, or ½ cup cooked spaghetti, macaroni or noodles.

Count 45 Calories for Each Fat Exchange

Fat is important in cooking, on vegetables and on breads. If your calorie budget allows use of fat, then count 45 calories for each exchange: 1 teaspoon butter or margarine (a small pat), 1 slice crisp bacon, 2 tablespoons light cream, 1 tablespoon heavy cream, 1 tablespoon French dressing, 1 teaspoon mayonnaise, 1 teaspoon oil or cooking fat or 6 small nuts or 5 small olives. Any one of these fat exchanges, whether used in cooking, on vegetables and meats, or as hors d'oeuvres, adds 45 calories to your day's total count.

CHAPTER 20

Practice
Using
Exchange Lists

IN ORDER TO familiarize yourself with the exchange list method of planning menus, try planning a few dinners of around 600 calories. Remember the three objectives: (1) nutritional balance, (2) calorie limitation, (3) enjoyment.

You may like this pattern. It uses 3 meat exchanges (3 x 75 calories equals 225 calories), 3 bread exchanges (3 x 70 calories equals 210 calories), 3 fat exchanges (3 x 45 calories equals 135 calories), 1 fruit exchange (40 calories), 2 vegetable List A exchanges (no calorie count). Total 610 calories.

DINNER MENU

(1) Celery and radishes, roast beef, pan gravy, mashed potatoes, buttered broccoli, lettuce and tomato salad, Zero dressing, ½ grapefruit, black coffee or tea (1 pat butter used in mashed potatoes and on broccoli).

(2) Small tomato juice, 2 medium lamb chops, sweet potato, asparagus, watercress and cucumber salad, French dressing, 1 pear, sponge cake, coffee or tea with light cream (1 pat butter used with sweet potatoes and asparagus).

(3) Celery and radishes, roast chicken, spaghetti with butter and cheese, beet greens, blueberries with light cream, coffee or tea (1 pat butter used in spaghetti and beet greens).

Breakfast Menus Easy with Exchange Lists

Now practice breakfast menus of about 400 calories using the exchange lists. Here are two variations of the same pattern: 1 fruit, 1 meat, 1 bread, 1 fat and 1 milk exchange. If you want a teaspoon of sugar in your coffee, add 16 calories; a rounded teaspoon of jelly on your toast, 30 more; a rounded teaspoon of marmalade, 55 calories.

BREAKFAST MENU

(1) An orange, 1 egg, 1 slice toast, 1 pat butter, 1 glass milk (8 ounces), coffee, tea—400 calories. With 1 teaspoon sugar and 1 teaspoon jelly, 446 calories.

(2) One-half grapefruit, bacon and egg, dry toast, milk (8 ounces), coffee, tea—400 calories. With 1 pat butter for toast, 445 calories. With 1 teaspoon marmalade instead of butter, 455 calories.

A few recipes are given to demonstrate how to use the exchange list, to make familiar dishes and still keep menus within your calorie budget. With a little practice, you can expand your list of exchange-list cooked dishes.

After you have memorized the six exchange lists given here, you can add more foods to each exchange. But be sure the food added contains not only the same number of calories as the other foods in the list, but also approximately the same number of grams of protein, carbohydrate and fat. Your best guides will be:

(1) *Composition of Foods, Raw, Processed, Prepared.* United States Department of Agriculture Handbook No. 8, Washington, D. C.

(2) Dr. Ruth M. Leverton, Institute of Home Economics, United States Department of Agriculture, Report of Research Project on Nutritional Values of Cooked Meat, 1957.

CHAPTER 21
The Six Basic Exchange Lists

THE EXCHANGE LISTS following are based on material in "Meal Planning with Exchange Lists," prepared by committees of the American Diabetes Association, Inc. and The American Dietetic Association in co-operation with the Chronic Disease Program, Public Health Service, Department of Health, Education and Welfare.

Your Meal Plan

This list of "Your Food for the Day," that your doctor or nutritionist gives you, will help you buy and plan your meals. Be sure to eat all the foods on your meal plan every day. You may take some of the meat and fat exchanges from one meal and add them to another. The rest of the foods should be taken as listed although a small amount may be saved to eat between meals. Do not eat more than is on your meal plan.

Make a daily menu plan within your calorie budget. Here is a graphic outline to use. It will save you the frustration of calorie counting and take self-consciousness out of your weight-reduction program.

Your Food for the Day

AMOUNT	KIND OF FOOD	CHOOSE FROM
——————————	Milk	List 1
Any Amount	Vegetable Exchanges A	List 2A
——————————	Vegetable Exchanges B	List 2B
——————————	Fruit Exchanges	List 3
——————————	Bread Exchanges	List 4
——————————	Meat Exchanges	List 5
——————————	Fat Exchanges	List 6

Divide this food as follows:

Your Meal Plan

BREAKFAST:

LUNCH OR SUPPER:

DINNER OR MAIN MEAL:

BEDTIME MEAL:

To measure your foods you will need a standard 8-ounce measuring cup, a teaspoon and a tablespoon. Keep the measures level. Most foods should be measured after they are cooked. Your foods may be prepared with the family meals but take your portion before extra fat or flour is added.

To season your food, you can use many things. Some suggestions are: chopped parsley, mint, garlic, onion, celery salt, nutmeg, mustard, cinnamon, pepper and other spices, lemon, saccharin, and vinegar. You may use all these foods freely.

Other foods that you do not need to measure are:

Coffee	Rennet Tablets
Tea	Pickles, sour
Clear Broth	Pickles, unsweetened dill
Bouillon (without fat)	Cranberries (unsweetened)
Gelatin (unsweetened)	Rhubarb (unsweetened)

You will also find many vegetables on List 2A that do not have much sugar. You can use them often.

Carbohydrate, Protein and Fat are the names of materials found in all foods. *Carbohydrates* (from breads, potatoes, fruits, etc.) give your body heat and energy. *Proteins* (from milk, meat, etc.) are needed for growth, building muscle and repairing body tissues. *Fats* (from butter, cream, margarine, etc.) are also used by your body for heat and energy.

Milk Exchanges—List 1

One exchange of milk contains 12 grams Carbohydrate, 8 grams Protein, 10 grams Fat and 170 Calories

Milk is one of our most important foods. You can use the milk on your meal plan to drink, in coffee, on cereal, or with other foods. You can use one type of milk instead of another. For example, you may use ½ cup evaporated milk in place of 1 cup of whole milk.

This list shows the different types of milk to use for one exchange.

Type of Milk	Amount to Use
Whole milk (plain or homogenized)	1 cup
* Skim milk	1 cup
Evaporated milk	½ cup
Powdered whole milk	¼ cup
* Powdered skim milk (non-fat dried milk)	¼ cup
Buttermilk (made from whole milk)	1 cup
* Buttermilk (made from skim milk)	1 cup

* You may wish to use skim milk or buttermilk made from skim milk instead of whole milk. Skim milk and buttermilk have the same food values as whole milk except they contain less fat. Add 2 fat exchanges to your meal when you use 1 cup of skim milk or buttermilk made from skim milk.

Vegetable Exchanges—List 2

All vegetables contain sugar but some have more sugar than others. The vegetables have been divided into three groups according to the amount of sugar they have:

List 2A vegetables have the smallest amount of sugar.

List 2B vegetables contain more sugar.

List 4 (see page 134) contains some vegetables which have a large amount of sugar.

You may serve vegetables plain or with part of the meat or fat exchange for seasoning. You may wish to use the vegetables, milk, and meat exchanges in your meal plan together. This way you can make soups, stews or other dishes.

For salads you may use mayonnaise or French dressing as your fat exchange. (For example, if you use 1 teaspoon of mayonnaise you would give up 1 teaspoon of butter.) Zero salad dressing (recipe pp. 140-141) may be used as desired.

VEGETABLE EXCHANGES A (Contain little Carbohydrate, Protein, or Calories)

You may eat as much of these vegetables raw as you wish, except tomatoes. (Limit tomatoes to one tomato or ½ cup tomato juice at a meal.) If these vegetables are cooked, you can use as much as one cup at a time. When you want more, you can use another cup of these vegetables in exchange for a List 2B vegetable.

Asparagus	Kale
* Broccoli	Mustard
Brussels Sprouts	Spinach
Cabbage	Turnip Greens
Cauliflower	Lettuce
Celery	Mushrooms
* Chicory	Okra
Cucumbers	* Pepper
* Escarole	Radishes
Eggplant	Sauerkraut
* Greens	String Beans, young
Beet Greens	Summer Squash
Chard	* Tomatoes
Collard	* Watercress
Dandelion	

* These vegetables contain a lot of Vitamin A.

VEGETABLE EXCHANGES B (Contain 7 grams Carbohydrate, 2 grams Protein and 35 Calories)

These vegetables contain more sugar than the vegetables in List 2A. You may use these vegetables raw or cooked.

Beets	Pumpkin
* Carrots	Rutabagas
Onions	* Squash, winter
Peas, green	Turnip

* These vegetables contain a lot of vitamin A.

Fruit Exchanges—List 3 One exchange of fruit contains 10 grams Carbohydrate and 40 Calories

Each exchange of fruit shown below contains about the same amount of sugar. Your meal plan will tell you how many exchanges you can have each day. You may use your fruit fresh, dried, cooked, canned or frozen as long as no sugar has been added. Look at the label on the can or package to be sure it says "unsweetened" or "no sugar added."

If dried fruits are used, the amount to take is small because they have a lot of sugar. You may take unsweetened fruit juice as part of the fruit in your meal plan. For variety, you can serve fruit as a salad or with unsweetened gelatin as a dessert.

This list shows the different amounts of fruits to use for one fruit exchange.

	AMOUNT TO USE
Apple (2″ diameter)	1 small
Applesauce	½ cup
Apricots, fresh	2 medium
Apricots, dried	4 halves
Banana	½ small
Blackberries	1 cup
Raspberries	1 cup
* Strawberries	1 cup
Blueberries	⅔ cup
* Canteloupe (6″ diameter)	¼

Cherries	10	large
Dates	2	
Figs, fresh	2	large
Figs, dried	1	small
* Grapefruit	½	small
* Grapefruit Juice	½	cup
Grapes	12	
Grape Juice	¼	cup
Honeydew Melon, medium	⅛	
Mango	½	small
* Orange	1	small
* Orange Juice	½	cup
Papaya	⅓	medium
Peach	1	medium
Pear	1	small
Pineapple	½	cup
Pineapple Juice	⅓	cup
Plums	2	medium
Prunes, dried	2	medium
Raisins	2	tablespoons
* Tangerine	1	large
Watermelon	1	cup

* These fruits are rich sources of vitamin C. Try to use one of them each day.

Bread Exchanges—List 4 One bread exchange contains 15 grams Carbohydrate, 2 grams Protein and 70 Calories

Whole-grain (dark) or enriched breads and cereals are good sources of iron and the B vitamins. Plan to use them often in your meal plan. They are better for you than white crackers, rice, or spaghetti that do not have the vitamins added. For variety, count potatoes, corn, lima beans, or cowpeas as a bread exchange.

Measure all the foods on the bread exchange list after they have been cooked.

Use these foods carefully because they have a lot of sugar.

For each bread exchange called for on your meal plan, choose any one item on the list below. For example:

½ cup cooked cereal will give you 1 bread exchange.

1 slice bread and 1 small potato will give you 2 bread exchanges.

1 slice bread and ½ cup cooked rice and ⅛ cup corn will give you 3 bread exchanges.

This list shows the different amounts of foods to use for one bread exchange.

	AMOUNT TO USE
Bread	1 slice
Biscuit, Roll (2″ diameter)	1
Muffin (2″ diameter)	1
Corn bread (1½″ cube)	1
Cereals, cooked	½ cup
Dry, flake and puff types	¾ cup
Rice, Grits, cooked	½ cup
Spaghetti, Noodles, cooked	½ cup
Macaroni, etc., cooked	½ cup
Crackers, graham (2½″ square)	2
Oyster (⅛ cup)	20
Saltines (2″ square)	5
Soda (2½″ square)	3
Round, Thin (1½″)	6
Flour	2½ tablespoons
Vegetables	
Beans & Peas, dried, cooked (lima, navy, split peas, cowpeas, etc.)	½ cup
Baked Beans, no pork	¼ cup
Corn	⅓ cup
Pop Corn	1 cup
Parsnips	⅔ cup
Potato, white	1 small
Potatoes, white, mashed	½ cup
Potatoes, sweet or Yams	¼ cup
Sponge Cake, plain (1½″ cube)	1
Ice cream (Omit 2 fat exchanges)	½ cup

Meat Exchanges—List 5 One meat exchange contains 7 grams Protein, 5 grams Fat and 75 Calories

You may have any kind of meat you wish. Cheese, eggs and peanut butter can be taken in place of meat for variety.

You may use the meat or fish, etc., that is prepared for the family as long as no fat or flour has been added. If you wish to fry your meat, you may do so with the fat you are allowed on your meal plan. Meat juices with the fat removed may be used with your meat or vegetables for added flavor.

It is important that you measure meat after it is cooked. Bones and extra fat should not be counted in the total weight. A 3-ounce serving of cooked meat is about equal to ¼ pound (4 ounces) of raw meat.

For each meat exchange called for on your meal plan choose any one item on the list below.

For example:

 1 egg will give you 1 meat exchange.
 1 ounce cheese and 1 ounce ham will give you 2 meat exchanges.
 1 egg and ¼ cup cottage cheese and 1 slice bologna will give you 3 meat exchanges.

This list shows the different amounts of foods to use for one meat exchange.

	AMOUNT TO USE
Meat & Poultry (medium fat) (Beef, Lamb, Pork, Liver, Chicken,etc.)	1 ounce
Cold Cuts (4½″ x ⅛″) (Salami, Minced Ham, Bologna, Liverwurst, Luncheon Loaf)	1 slice
Frankfurter (8-9 per pound)	1
Egg	1
* Peanut Butter	2 tablespoons
Fish: Haddock, etc.	1 ounce

Salmon, Tuna, Crab, Lobster	¼ cup
Shrimp, Clams, Oysters, etc.	5 small
Sardines	3 medium
Cheese, cheddar type	1 ounce
Cottage	¼ cup

* Limit peanut butter to one exchange a day unless the carbohydrate in it is allowed for in your meal plan.

Here are some examples of foods that are equal to three meat exchanges.

¼ cup cottage cheese, 1 egg, 1 ounce ham
1 pork chop (3 ounces) large omelet (3 eggs)
2 lamb chops (3 ounces) roast chicken (3 ounces)

1 small fish (3 ounces)
2 meat balls (3 ounces) roast beef (3 ounces) broiled liver (3 ounces)

Fat Exchanges—List 6 One fat exchange contains 5 grams Fat and 45 Calories

All fat foods are high in calories. Too much fat or too much of any food may cause you to gain weight. A person with diabetes should try to reach his ideal weight. If he weighs too much his diabetes will be harder to control.

Use the foods on this list only as allowed on your meal plan.

You may use your fat exchanges in preparing such foods as vegetables and meats. For example, if you use a teaspoon of fat to fry an egg give up one fat exchange.

For each fat exchange called for on your meal plan choose any one item on the list below.

For example:

1 teaspoon butter will give you 1 fat exchange.
1 teaspoon margarine and 1 slice bacon will give you 2 fat exchanges.

This list shows the different foods to use for one fat exchange.

	AMOUNT TO USE
Butter or Margarine	1 teaspoon
Bacon, crisp	1 slice
Cream, light	2 tablespoons
Cream, heavy	1 tablespoon
Cream Cheese	1 tablespoon
Avocado (4″ diameter)	⅛
French Dressing	1 tablespoon
Mayonnaise	1 teaspoon
Oil or Cooking Fat	1 teaspoon
Nuts	6 small
Olives	5 small

Recipes

These recipes follow the pattern you will find in any cookbook. There are examples here to show you how you may combine foods from different lists. In this way you can make a variety of hot dishes and desserts to fit into your meal plan.

Beside each recipe you will find the exchanges that are used. This will help you to know what to leave off when you use the recipe.

Your family may enjoy these recipes too. You can increase the recipe by the number to be served. Take your exact portion.

LEMON GELATIN (May be used in any amount)

1 teaspoon unflavored gelatin   1 tablespoon lemon juice
2 tablespoons cold water   ½ cup water

Put cold water in top of double boiler, add gelatin, let stand 10 minutes at room temperature. Place pan over boiling water to dissolve gelatin. If you wish you may add ¼ grain of saccharin to flavor. Remove from stove. Add lemon juice and ½ cup of water. Chill. To make *Coffee Gelatin* omit lemon juice and use ½ cup coffee in place of ½ cup water.

ORANGE GELATIN (1 Serving equals 1 Fruit from List 3)

Use ½ cup orange juice in place of water in recipe for lemon gelatin.

PINEAPPLE GELATIN (1 Serving *equals* 1 Fruit from List 3)

| 1 teaspoon unflavored gelatin | 1 tablespoon lemon juice |
| ¼ cup cold water | ⅓ cup pineapple juice |

FRUIT GELATIN—I (1 Serving *equals* 1 Fruit from List 3)

One serving of any fruit from List 3 may be added to lemon gelatin, such as ½ small banana

FRUIT GELATIN—II (1 Serving *equals* 2 Fruits from List 3)

One serving of any fruit from List 3 may be added to orange or pineapple gelatin.

FRUIT ICE (1 Serving *equals* 1 Fruit from List 3)

½ cup orange juice *or*	1 egg white
⅓ cup pineapple juice	
1 tablespoon lemon juice	½ cup water

Combine fruit juice and water and freeze. Stir mixture often while freezing. When almost hard fold in one stiffly beaten egg white.

FRESH FRUIT CUP (1 Serving *equals* 1 Fruit from List 3)

Any fruits in List 3 may be combined to make a fruit cup. One-half cup of mixed fruits equals 1 serving.

Example

Orange, Grapefruit, Pineapple	Peach, Orange, Blackberries
Apple, Grapefruit, Strawberries	Grapes, Orange, Melon
Melon, Grapefruit, Banana	

CANNING FRUIT WITHOUT SUGAR (1 Serving *equals* 1 Fruit from List 3)

Any fruit—peaches, pears, etc., may be canned at home by following the usual directions for canning except that you omit the sugar. Can fruit in its own juice with enough water added to fill the jar. You will find directions in any cookbook for the amount of time to steam the fruit. The fruit will keep all right if the can is properly sealed.

BAKED CUSTARD (1 Serving *equals* ½ cup Milk and 1 Meat Exchange)

| 1 egg | Few grains salt | ⅛ teaspoon vanilla |
| ½ cup milk | | Sprinkle of nutmeg |

Beat the egg slightly; stir in milk, salt and vanilla. If you wish, add ¼ grain saccharin to flavor. Pour into a custard cup and sprinkle with nutmeg. Set in pan of hot water and bake in a moderate oven (350°) for about 45 minutes.

Other flavors, such as almond, lemon, orange or maple, may be used in place of vanilla.

CHEESE FONDUE (1 Serving *equals* 1 Bread Exchange and 2 Meat Exchanges and 1 cup Milk)

1 egg
1 cup milk
Salt, pepper, chopped parsley and onion

1 slice bread, cubed
¼ cup cheese, diced (1 oz.)

Beat the egg, add milk, bread, cheese and seasoning. Bake in a moderate oven (350°) until firm in the center, about 20 or 30 minutes.

In place of cheese ¼ cup (1 oz.) of chopped ham, chicken, tuna fish or salmon may be used.

MEAT STEW (1 Serving *equals* 2 or 3 Meat Exchanges and 1 Bread Exchange and 1 Serving Vegetable from List 2B and 1 Fat Exchange)

1 teaspoon fat
½ cup mixed vegetables, list 2B
(carrots, peas, onions)

2 or 3 oz. meat, cubed
1 small potato
Salt and pepper to taste

Brown meat in fat. Add 1 cup water, salt and pepper, and a few celery leaves for seasoning. Simmer slowly until meat is tender. Add ½ cup vegetables, List 2B, and any additional vegetables from List 2A, if desired. Cut potato into quarters and add. Cook for 30 minutes or until vegetables are done.

BAKED CHICKEN AND RICE (1 Serving *equals* 1 Bread Exchange and 1 or 2 Meat Exchanges)

½ cup cooked rice
¼ or ½ cup diced chicken
(1 or 2 oz.)

¼ cup clear broth
Salt and pepper

Chopped parsley, onions, celery, mushrooms, green pepper, pimento, *or* tomatoes may be added for variety, if desired.

Combine the above ingredients and place in dish. Bake in a moderate oven until brown.

In place of rice you may use noodles or spaghetti. For the chicken you may use any type of meat or fish, such as lamb, ham, tuna or shrimp.

FISH CHOWDER (1 Serving *equals* 1 Fat Exchange and 1 Bread Exchange and 1 or 2 Meat Exchanges and 1 cup Milk)

1 teaspoon fat	¼ or ½ cup cooked fish (1 or 2
½ small onion, chopped	oz.)
1 small potato, sliced	1 cup milk
Salt and pepper	

Cook fish in salted water. Melt fat in saucepan, brown the onion. Add cooked fish, sliced potato, ½ cup water in which fish was cooked. Cover and cook for 15 minutes until potatoes are tender. Add milk and seasonings.

VEGETABLE SOUP (1 Serving *equals* 1 Vegetable from List 2B)

1 cup meat stock *or* bouillon cube and 1 cup water	¼ cup cabbage, shredded
	1 stalk celery, diced
½ cup mixed vegetables: carrots, peas	¼ cup tomato juice
	Salt and pepper
½ small onion, chopped	

Prepare vegetables and add to broth. Boil together until vegetables are just tender, about 20 minutes.

POTATO SALAD A (1 Serving *equals* 1 Bread Exchange)

½ cup cooked potato, diced	1 or 2 tablespoons Zero salad
Salt, pepper, chopped onion, celery, parsley, green pepper, as desired.	dressing

Combine ingredients and serve.

POTATO SALAD B (1 Serving *equals* 1 Fat Exchange and 1 Bread Exchange)

Use same recipe as Potato Salad A except that 1 teaspoon of mayonnaise may be used in place of Zero salad dressing.

POTATO SALAD C (1 Serving *equals* 1 Bread Exchange and 1 Meat Exchange and 1 Fat Exchange *if desired*)

1 hard-cooked egg, sliced, may be added to recipe for Potato Salad A or B.

¼ cup (1 oz.) diced ham, bologna or frankfurt, or 5 small shrimp may be used in place of egg.

ZERO SALAD DRESSING (May be used in any amount)

½ cup tomato juice	1 tablespoon onion, finely
2 tablespoons lemon juice or vinegar	chopped
	Salt and pepper

Chopped parsley or green pepper, horseradish, or mustard, etc., may be added, if desired.

Combine ingredients in a jar with a tightly fitted top. Shake well before using.

ITALIAN SPAGHETTI (1 Serving *equals* 1 or 2 Meat Exchanges and 1 or 2 Bread Exchanges and 1 Fat Exchange)

1 teaspoon fat	Salt, pepper
2 tablespoons tomato paste	½ cup tomatoes
½ small onion, chopped	1 or 2 oz. hamburg
¼ cup water	½ cup cooked spaghetti

Brown the onion, hamburg and fat. Add the tomato paste, water and tomatoes. Allow to simmer gently one or more hours. If needed, add more water. Serve on ½ or 1 cup cooked spaghetti. 1 or 2 teaspoons grated cheese may be used.

MACARONI AND CHEESE (1 Serving *equals* 1 Bread Exchange and 1 or 2 Meat Exchanges and 1/4 cup Milk)

½ cup cooked macaroni
¼ or ½ cup diced cheese (1 or 2 oz.)
¼ cup milk
Salt, pepper, dash of mustard

Cook cheese and milk together in double boiler until smooth. Add macaroni and mix well. Bake in moderate oven about 20 minutes, or until brown.

In place of macaroni you may use ½ cup cooked rice, noodles or spaghetti.

MIXED VEGETABLE SALAD (May be used in any amount)

Any combination of vegetables from List 2A may be used, such as:

1. Lettuce, cucumber, celery, green pepper
2. Chicory, tomato, radish
3. Lettuce, parsley, raw cauliflower, tomato
4. Escarole, tomato, cucumber
5. Cabbage, celery, green pepper
6. Lettuce, watercress, cucumber
7. Lettuce, raw spinach, radish

Salad may be combined with Zero salad dressing, French dressing, or Mayonnaise, depending upon fat allowed in your meal plan.

PART VII

SEVEN-DAY
LOW-CALORIE
DIETS USING
MEAT, BREAD,
CEREALS AND
DAIRY PRODUCTS
LIBERALLY

CHAPTER 22

High-Protein,
Moderate-Fat Diets

THESE high-protein, moderate-fat menus contain at least two large servings of meat a day, plus either meat or eggs at breakfast.

Because meat plays so important a part in most normal American eating habits, it is a basic food in our cultural pattern. Therefore, for many people it must be included in any long-term weight-reducing program.

According to Charlotte M. Young, Ph.D., professor of Medical Nutrition, Cornell University, "There is never a time when the 'staying' or 'stick to the ribs' quality of meat is more important or more appreciated than by the consumer of a low-calorie reducing diet."

Gives Dieter Sense of Well-being

She explains that the high-protein, moderate-fat diet has been shown in the experiences of many researchers, as well as her own, to lead to a greater sense of well-being on the part of the dieter, to less between-meal hunger, to less fatigue and to a greater willingness to continue on the diet than is found with lower protein diets.

The reason for the greater satiety value is not clear, but it does *not* appear to be related to blood sugar levels. The use of more fat in the diet has two psychological advantages: an encouraging initial rapid loss of weight and a remarkable steady loss of weight in most cases with little evidence of plateauing, which can be so discouraging to the patient.

High-Protein, Moderate-Fat Seven-Day Diet Series

PREPARED BY:

Rita Campbell, M.S., University of Manitoba; member, American Dietetic Association; American Public Health Association and Institute of Food Technologists.

Frances Hall, B.S., University of Washington; member, American Dietetic Association.

FIRST DAY

1,200-Calorie Diet   *1,500-Calorie Diet*

BREAKFAST

Orange juice (4 ounces)
Poached eggs (2)
Toast (1 slice)
Butter *or* Margarine (1 pat)
Coffee *or* Tea (if desired)

LUNCH

Braised lamb chop (3 ounces)   add
Broccoli (⅓ cup)   Enriched bread (1 slice)
Lettuce-tomato salad   Butter *or* Margarine (1 pat)
Milk, non-fat (1 cup)
Coffee *or* Tea (if desired)

DINNER

Blade pot roast (3½ ounces)   add
Green beans (½ cup)   Blade pot roast (1 ounce)
Butter *or* Margarine (1 pat)   Boiled potato (1 medium)
Peaches (½ cup), water-packed
  or fresh without sugar
Milk, non-fat (1 cup)
Coffee *or* Tea (if desired)

NOTES: *The pat of butter at dinner could be used half on broccoli at lunch and the other on beans at dinner.*
  The cup of non-fat milk at dinner can be used later for bedtime snack, if desired

One pat of butter as used in these menus is 1½ teaspoons, which is equal to 50 calories. There are 16 pats in each quarter of a pound, or 64 pats in a pound.

SECOND DAY

1,200-Calorie Diet   *1,500-Calorie Diet*

BREAKFAST

Grapefruit (½)   add
Soft-cooked eggs (2)   Sausage links (2)
Toast (1 slice)
Butter *or* Margarine (1 pat)
Coffee *or* Tea (if desired)

LUNCH

Ground beef patty (3 ounces)   add
Beets (½ cup)   Enriched or whole-wheat bread
Mayonnaise (1 tablespoon)   (1 slice)
Cole slaw (½ cup)   Butter *or* Margarine (1 pat)
Milk, non-fat (1 cup)
Coffee *or* Tea (if desired)

DINNER

Tomato juice (3 ounces)   add
Baked salmon *or* Baked ham   Baked salmon *or* Baked ham
  (3½ ounces)   (1 ounce)
Spinach (½ cup)
Butter *or* Margarine (1 pat)
Carrot sticks (½ carrot)
Milk, non-fat (1 cup)
Coffee *or* Tea (if desired)

NOTE: *The cup of non-fat milk at dinner can be used later for bedtime snack if desired.*

THIRD DAY

1,200-Calorie Diet   *1,500-Calorie Diet*

BREAKFAST

Orange slices
Poached eggs (2)

Toast (1 slice)
Butter *or* Margarine (1 pat)
Coffee *or* Tea (if desired)

LUNCH

Fried liver with bacon (2 slices)   add
Green peas (½ cup)   Enriched or whole-wheat bread
Lettuce wedge (⅙ head)   (1 slice)
French dressing (1 tablespoon)   Butter *or* Margarine (1 pat)
Milk, non-fat (1 cup)
Coffee *or* Tea (if desired)

DINNER

Roast leg of lamb   add
  (3½ ounces)   Roast leg of lamb (1 ounce)
Carrots (⅓ cup)   Mashed potatoes (½ cup)
Butter *or* Margarine (1 pat)
Cabbage-pineapple salad
  (½ cup)
Milk, non-fat (1 cup)
Coffee *or* Tea (if desired)

NOTE: *The cup of non-fat milk at dinner can be used later for bedtime snack, if desired.*

FOURTH DAY

1,200-Calorie Diet   *1,500-Calorie Diet*

BREAKFAST

Orange juice (4 ounces)
Soft-cooked eggs (2)
Toast (1 slice)
Butter *or* Margarine (1 pat)
Coffee *or* Tea (if desired)

LUNCH

Luncheon meat salad (3 ounces   add
  meat with ¼ cup celery and   Whole-wheat bread (1 slice)
  green pepper)   Butter *or* Margarine (1 pat)

Stewed tomatoes (½ cup)
Milk, non-fat (1 cup)
Coffee *or* Tea (if desired)

DINNER

Smoked shoulder butt
  (3½ ounces)
Cabbage (½ cup)
Butter *or* Margarine (1 pat)
Grapefruit sections unsweetened
  or fresh without sugar (½
  cup)
Milk, non-fat (1 cup)
Coffee *or* Tea (if desired)

add

Smoked shoulder butt
  (1 ounce)
Boiled potato (1 small)

NOTE: *The cup of non-fat milk at dinner can be used later for bedtime snack if desired.*

FIFTH DAY

1,200-Calorie Diet   *1,500-Calorie Diet*

BREAKFAST

Grapefruit juice (4 ounces)
Cereal (unsweetened) (1 cup)
  with milk, non-fat (½ cup)
Toast (1 slice)
Butter *or* Margarine (1 pat)
Coffee *or* Tea (if desired)

add

Sausage links (2)

LUNCH

Tomato juice (3 ounces)
Beef brisket (3 ounces)
Green beans (½ cup)
Lettuce wedge (⅛ head)
Milk, non-fat (1 cup)
Coffee *or* Tea (if desired)

add

Enriched or whole-wheat bread
  (1 slice)
Butter *or* Margarine (1 pat)

DINNER

Ground beef patty (3½ ounces)
Cauliflower (½ cup)

add

Ground beef patty (1 ounce)

Butter *or* Margarine (1 pat)
Carrot sticks (½ carrot)
Vanilla ice cream (¼ pint)
Milk, non-fat (1 cup)
Coffee *or* Tea (if desired)

NOTE: *The cup of non-fat milk at dinner can be used later for bedtime snack if desired.*

SIXTH DAY

1,200-Calorie Diet   *1,500-Calorie Diet*

BREAKFAST

Orange juice (4 ounces)   add
Canadian-style bacon (3 slices)   Egg (1)
Toast (1 slice)
Butter *or* Margarine (1 pat)
Coffee *or* Tea (if desired)

LUNCH

Pork chop (3 ounces)   add
Squash (½ cup)   Enriched or whole-wheat bread
Apple-celery salad on lettuce (⅛   (1 slice)
   cup apple, ¼ cup celery)   Butter *or* Margarine (1 pat)
Milk, non-fat (1 cup)
Coffee *or* Tea (if desired)

DINNER

Tomato juice (2 ounces)   add
Roast beef (3½ ounces)   Tomato juice (2 ounces)
Wax beans (½ cup)   Roast beef (1 ounce)
Butter *or* Margarine (1 pat)
Celery sticks
Milk, non-fat (1 cup)
Coffee *or* Tea (if desired)

NOTE: *The cup of non-fat milk at dinner can be used later for bedtime snack if desired.*

SEVENTH DAY

1,200-Calorie Diet   *1,500-Calorie Diet*

BREAKFAST

Grapefruit sections (½ cup)
Scrambled eggs (2)
Toast (1 slice)
Butter *or* Margarine (1 pat)
Coffee *or* Tea (if desired)

LUNCH

Sirloin steak (3 ounces)   add
Boiled onions (½ cup)   Enriched or whole-wheat bread
Cottage cheese and peach salad   (1 slice)
Milk, non-fat (1 cup)   Butter *or* Margarine (1 pat)
Coffee *or* Tea (if desired)

DINNER

Roast turkey *or* Roast pork loin   add
   (3½ ounces)   Roast turkey *or* Roast pork loin
Carrots (½ cup)   (1 ounce)
Butter *or* Margarine (1 pat)   Mashed potatoes (½ cup)
Sliced tomatoes (1 small)
French dressing (½ tablespoon)
Milk, non-fat (1 cup)
Coffee *or* Tea (if desired)

NOTE: *The cup of non-fat milk at dinner can be used later for bedtime snack if desired.*

CHAPTER 23

Milk and
Dairy Products Used

MILK and dairy products such as cheese, ice cream, etc., play an important role in the American diet, both nutritionally and culturally. In no other country is the overall standard and supply so high.

Because dairy products are the most highly concentrated source of calcium in available dietary form, some use of them is essential in all balanced diets, especially for children, teenagers and pregnant and nursing women.

Milk Emotionally Important to Many Dieters

The following seven-day reducing diets include larger amounts of milk and dairy foods than most. Nevertheless, they are nutritionally balanced and have been prepared by one of the most distinguished nutritionists in the country. For the dieter whose cultural pattern has from childhood included liberal amounts of dairy products, these special diets will help him lose weight without a feeling of being deprived of familiar foods.

Seven-Day 1,400- and 1,800-Calorie Diets
with Liberal Use of Dairy Foods

Based on research at Michigan State University under direction of Margaret A. Ohlson, Ph.D., director of nutrition, State University of Iowa Hospitals; formerly head of Department of Foods and Nutrition, Michigan State University.

How to Follow the Diet Plan

Eat the three meals at well-spaced intervals every day—Sundays and holidays. The full breakfast probably is the most important part in the success of the plan. You may have coffee and tea, unsweetened, in any amount your doctor suggests. Add to it part of your milk or a little whipped cream if you wish. Consommé and lemon juice may be used at will. Alcoholic and sweetened beverages are not included in this reducing diet. Cook meat any way desired. Use the drippings, including the fat, unthickened. These are recommended to season vegetables. Use fruits unsweetened or canned in light syrup. All portions listed are for cooked or ready-to-eat foods, without bone or waste.

Minor variations that do not alter the basic plan may be made in your meals to fit individual situations.

Meats can be exchanged to suit taste. Avoid salted meats, as ham or bacon, if your body tissues tend to hold water in excess. A 4-ounce serving of cooked meat, without bone, is about 4 inches by 3 inches by 1 inch, usually ⅓ pound or more uncooked. Cheese may be used for part of a meat serving. A medium slice or a 1-inch cube of cheese or 2 tablespoons of cottage cheese is about 1 ounce.

More butter may be allowed by using non-fat milk. The diet is planned with whole milk or the equivalent. Three-fourths cup of non-fat milk plus ¾ medium pat of butter equals ¾ cup whole milk (6 ounces). Cut butter 12 pats to quarter pound for ⅓ ounce medium-sized pats.

Foods in these groups can be exchanged for each other *except at breakfast:*

Fruits: grapefruit, orange, melon, berries, black cherries, pears, apricots, peaches, grapes, pineapple, apples.

Vegetables: broccoli, asparagus, beets, green beans, cabbage, Brussels sprouts, tomatoes, greens, summer squash.

Vegetables: potatoes, winter squash, peas, corn, green lima beans.

About 1,400 Calories a Day

BREAKFAST EACH DAY

Grapefruit	½ medium
or	
Orange	1 small
or	
Citrus fruit juice	½ cup (4 ounces)
Eggs	2 (cooked as you please)
Bread	1 thin slice
Butter	1 medium pat (use part for eggs)
Milk, whole	1 small glass (¾ cup or 6 ounces)

LUNCH 1

Pork chop	1 large (4 ounces)
Broccoli	⅔ cup (3½ ounces)
Milk, whole	1 6-ounce glass

DINNER 1

Hamburger	2 medium (4 ounces)
Potato	1 small (3 ounces)
Butter,	½ medium pat
Grapefruit sections	½ cup (3½ ounces)
Milk, whole	1 6-ounce glass

LUNCH 2

Lamb patties	2 medium (4 ounces)
Fruit salad:	
lettuce	2 large or 3 small leaves
pears	2 medium halves (3½ ounces)
Milk, whole	1 6-ounce glass

DINNER 2

Grilled steak, cube or other	4 ounces
Green beans	⅔ cup (3½ ounces)
Applesauce, unsweetened	½ cup (3½ ounces)
Milk, whole	1 6-ounce glass

LUNCH 3

Meat loaf, large serving	4 ounces
Tomato-cottage cheese salad	
lettuce	2 large or 3 small leaves
tomato	1 medium
cottage cheese	½ cup
Milk, whole	1 6-ounce glass

DINNER 3

Roast beef	4 ounces
Squash, yellow	½ cup (3½ ounces)
Butter	medium pat
Berries	⅔ cup (3½ ounces)
Milk, whole	1 6-ounce glass

LUNCH 4

Hamburger	2 medium (4 ounces)
Asparagus	6-8 spears (3½ ounces)
Milk, whole	1 6-ounce glass

DINNER 4

Pork roast	4 ounces
Beets	⅔ cup (3½ ounces)
Apricots, canned	4 halves, ½ cup (3½ ounces)
Milk, whole	1 6-ounce glass

LUNCH 5

Fish salad:	
salmon	¾ cup (4 ounces)
celery	1 stalk
mayonnaise	1 tablespoon
Green beans	⅔ cup (3½ ounces)
Butter	medium pat
Milk, whole	1 6-ounce glass

DINNER 5

Broiled fish	4 ounces
Baked potato, small	3½ ounces
Butter	medium pat
Milk, whole	1 6-ounce glass

LUNCH 6

Cold roast pork	4 ounces
Tossed salad	1 cup (3½ ounces)
French dressing	1 teaspoon
Milk, whole	1 6-ounce glass

DINNER 6

Steak	4 ounces
Creamed potatoes	½ cup (3½ ounces)
Peaches	2 medium halves, ½ cup (3½ ounces)
Milk, whole	1 6-ounce glass

LUNCH 7

Meat sandwich:	
meat loaf	4 ounces
enriched bread	2 very thin slices (1 ounce)
butter	½ medium pat
Apple	1 medium (5 ounces)
Milk, whole	1 6-ounce glass

DINNER 7

Roast chicken	4-5 ounces
Peas	⅔ cup (3½ ounces)
Butter	½ medium pat
Lettuce salad	¼ medium head
French dressing	1 teaspoon
Milk, whole	1 6-ounce glass

NOTE: *Coffee or tea without sugar can be used at each meal. Use part of day's milk allotment with beverage, if desired.*

About 1,800 Calories a Day

Add to the basic 1,400-calorie diet about ½ slice enriched bread
and ½ pat of butter.

One or more ounces meat or cheese.

One serving vegetable, fruit or salad.

Three-quarters cup milk or a milk dessert such as ice cream or
custard.

CHAPTER 24

Bread and Cereals
Used in Diets

IF A SLICE of bread with your meals is important to you, even though you want to lose weight, go ahead and enjoy it. Enriched bread is good food. It is a fine source of thiamine, along with liver and pork, and adds many nutrients to a balanced diet.

Breakfast cereals, either whole-grained or reconstituted, are also important nutritionally. They are low in fat content. A cereal breakfast consisting of fruit or fruit juice, cereal with milk, and toast, with beverage, will give the dieter a moderately low-calorie breakfast with high nutritional value.

The following 1,500-calorie and 1,800-calorie seven-day diets have been planned for those dieters who are happier with bread and cereals in their meals. They include many kinds of bread and also several sandwiches, hot and cold cereal, cake and cookies. Yet they are nutritionally balanced and within the calorie budget.

Note the following "Menu-way to Follow," a guide to the types and amounts of foods used in the seven-day diets. It is a working plan to help you plan your own balanced menus within the calorie limitations, using bread and cereals liberally.

A Menu-Way to Follow

BREAKFAST	1,500 Calories	1,800 Calories
Fruit *or* Juice	1 serving	1 serving
Egg *or* ½ to ¾ cup Cereal with scant ½ cup milk	1	1

158

Bacon	None	2 strips, drained
Enriched or whole-grain bread or rolls	1 slice	2 slices
Butter *or* Margarine	1 teaspoon	2 teaspoons
Coffee *or* Tea	As desired	As desired

LUNCHEON

Meat *or* Vegetable bouillon *or* Selections from list of "free foods"	As desired	As desired
Sandwich	1	1
Lean meat, egg, fish, cheese	1 serving	1 serving
Enriched or whole-grain bread or rolls	2 slices	2 slices
Butter *or* Margarine	1 teaspoon	1 teaspoon
Vegetable as salad *or* Relish	As desired	As desired
* Dessert	1 serving	1 serving
Milk	1 cup, non-fat	1 cup, whole

DINNER

Bouillon, as above	As desired	As desired
Lean meat	1 serving	1 serving
Potato *or* alternate	1 serving	1 serving
Vegetable. Let it be deep green or yellow at least every other day.	1 serving	1 serving
Vegetable salad	As desired	As desired
Enriched or whole-grain bread or rolls	1 slice	1 slice
Butter *or* Margarine	1 teaspoon	1 teaspoon

* Dessert	1 serving	1 serving
Milk	1 cup, non-fat	1 cup, whole
† Bonus	1 each day	1 each day

* Select a fruit at one meal; at another, choose a dessert which combines good foods, foods such as eggs, milk, enriched flour, etc. Examples are plain cake or cookies, cupcake, sponge or angel cake, ice cream or sherbet, custards, bread puddings without raisins or nuts.

† Bonus, part and parcel of the menu-way, allows you to select a food you particularly like or want to like. To vary your milk quota, for example, your bonus may be an addition to dessert or camembert, cheddar, or other cheese, which can substitute for one serving of milk. Or the bonus might be added as we have added them in the menus to follow: a sauce with meat or vegetable, bacon strips, an extra fruit to top off ice cream or cake. Only when the menu-way (pp. 158-159) has been followed—to be sure of needed nutrients—can the bonus be a before-dinner drink.

One nutrient most apt to be shorted in any food plan is thiamine. Reducing menus must be carefully checked to see that these good sources of thiamine are included often: liver, pork, enriched and whole-grain bread and cereal.

Seven-Day 1,500- and 1,800-Calorie Diets with Liberal Use of Breads and Cereals

PREPARED BY:

Mary Ellis, M.S., Teachers College, Columbia University; member, American Dietetic Association.
Norine Condon, M.S., Ohio State University; member, American Dietetic Association.

Sunday

BRUNCH	*1,500 Calories*	*1,800 Calories*
Chilled tomato juice with lemon slice	Scant ½ cup	Scant ½ cup
Egg, poached in milk, on enriched toast	1 egg	2 eggs
	2 tablespoons milk	2 tablespoons milk
	1 slice bread	1 slice bread
Coffee *or* Tea	As desired	As desired

DINNER

Rib of beef au jus	3 slices (3x2¼x ¼-inch)	3 slices (3x2¼x ¼-inch)
with mushrooms	4 large	4 large
Oven-browned potato	1 small	1 medium
5-minute caraway cabbage	½ cup cabbage	½ cup cabbage
Rutabaga wedges	As desired	As desired
Hot cloverleaf roll	1 roll	1 roll
Butter	1 teaspoon	1 teaspoon
Peaches and plums with kirsch	1 serving	1 serving
Milk	1 cup	1 cup, whole

SUPPER

Oxtail soup	1 serving	1 serving
Celery root with green onions	4-6 slices celery root, 3 onions	4-6 slices celery root, 3 onions
Dark rye bread and butter sandwich	1 slice bread, 1 teaspoon butter	2 slices bread, 1 teaspoon butter
Strawberry sundae,	1 serving	1 serving
Vanilla ice cream	⅛ quart	⅛ quart
Strawberries, fresh or frozen	½ cup	½ cup
Milk	1 cup	1 cup, whole

Monday

BREAKFAST	*1,500 Calories*	*1,800 Calories*
Orange slices with mint sprigs	1 small orange	1 medium orange
Cooked oat cereal	¾ cup	¾ cup
with whole milk	Scant ½ cup	Scant ½ cup
Raisin toast	1 slice	2 slices
Butter	1 teaspoon	2 teaspoons
Coffee *or* Tea	As desired	As desired

LUNCHEON

Bouillon with minced leek atop	As desired	As desired
Liverwurst sandwich	1 sandwich	1 sandwich
liverwurst	2 slices (¼x3-inch diameter)	2 slices (¼x3-inch diameter)
whole-wheat bread	2 slices	2 slices
butter	½ teaspoon	1 teaspoon
Tomato wedges	1 small tomato	1 medium tomato
Chilled melon	½ of 4½-inch melon	½ of 4½-inch melon
Milk	1 cup, non-fat	1 cup, whole

DINNER

Broiled chicken (¼ of 2-pound chicken)	1 serving	1 serving
Brown rice	½ cup	½ cup
Asparagus spears	5-6 stalks	5-6 stalks
Romaine and watercress (or other greens)	As desired	As desired
Hot cloverleaf roll	1 small	1 small
Butter	½ teaspoon	1 teaspoon
Angel cake with low-calorie vanilla pudding with grated coconut and grated lemon rind.	1 serving	1 serving
Milk	1 cup, non-fat	1 cup, whole

Tuesday

BREAKFAST

	1,500 Calories	1,800 Calories
Grapefruit juice	Scant ½ cup	Scant ½ cup
Bran flakes	¾ cup	¾ cup
with whole milk	½ cup	½ cup
Hot, plain breakfast roll	1 small	1 small
Butter	1 teaspoon	1 teaspoon
Coffee *or* Tea	As desired	As desired

LUNCHEON

Chef's salad with ham and Swiss cheese julienne	1 serving	1 serving
Hard roll	1 average	1 average
Butter	1 teaspoon	1 teaspoon
Custard pie	⅛ medium	⅛ medium
Coffee *or* Tea	As desired	As desired

DINNER

Bourbon on the rocks	None	1 ounce bourbon
Roast leg of lamb	2 slices (3x3¼x ⅛-inch)	2 slices (3x3¼x ⅛-inch)
with		
mint sauce	As desired	As desired
Baked potato	1 small (2½-inch diameter)	1 medium
with		
churned buttermilk	Scant ½ cup	Scant ½ cup
crisp bacon bits	None	2 tablespoons
Green beans with carrot rings	1 serving	1 serving
Curly spinach, tossed with cottage cheese	As desired 1 rounded tablespoon	As desired 1 rounded tablespoon
Enriched bread	1 slice	1 slice
Butter	1 teaspoon	1 teaspoon
Grapes	1 bunch, 22-24 grapes	1 bunch, 22-24 grapes
Coffee *or* Tea	As desired	As desired

Wednesday

BREAKFAST

	1,500 Calories	*1,800 Calories*
Fresh cinnamon applesauce	1 medium apple	1 medium apple
Scrambled egg	1 serving	1 serving
Whole-wheat roll	1 roll	1 roll
Butter	1 teaspoon	1 teaspoon
Coffee *or* Tea	As desired	As desired

LUNCHEON

Chicken bouillon	As desired	As desired
Open-faced shrimp sandwich	1 sandwich	2 sandwiches
rye bread	1 slice	2 slices
sweet butter	1 teaspoon	2 teaspoons
shrimp	4-6 large, or 8-10 small	8-12 large or 16-20 small
horseradish	As desired	As desired
Pickled beets on watercress	2 small beets	2 small beets
Chilled apricots	4 halves, juice-pack	4 halves, juice-pack
	2 tablespoons juice	2 tablespoons juice
Oatmeal cookie	1 large cookie	1 large cookie
Milk	1 glass, non-fat	1 glass, whole

DINNER

Beef (¼ pound round, cut in strips, marinated in 1½ tablespoons soy sauce, 1 teaspoon salad oil and strips of green pepper and tomato)	1 serving	1 serving
Fordhook lima beans	3 rounded tablespoons	3 rounded tablespoons
Hot enriched Vienna bread with herb butter	1 thick slice	1 thick slice
	1 teaspoon	1 teaspoon
Large salad bowl with seasoned salt	1 serving	1 serving
Lime sherbet with fresh or water-pack blueberries	½ cup	½ cup
	2 tablespoons	2 tablespoons
Milk	1 glass, non-fat	1 glass, whole

Thursday

BREAKFAST

	1,500 Calories	*1,800 Calories*
Fruit compote	1 serving	1 serving
prunes	2 prunes	2 prunes

apricots	3 apricots	3 apricots
or Banana	1 medium	1 medium
Wheat flakes with	¾ cup	¾ cup
whole milk	Scant ½ cup	Scant ½ cup
Breakfast roll	1 roll	None
Cinnamon bun with raisins	None	1 bun
Butter	1 teaspoon	1 teaspoon
Coffee *or* Tea	As desired	As desired

LUNCHEON

Celery bouillon	As desired	As desired
Sliced lamb sandwich	1 sandwich	1 sandwich
enriched bread	2 slices	2 slices
butter	1 teaspoon	1 teaspoon
cold sliced lamb	2 slices (3x3¼x ⅛-inch)	2 slices (3x3¼x ⅛-inch)
Pickled peach slices	½ fresh or juice-pack peach	½ fresh or juice-pack peach
Cauliflower florets	2-3 florets	2-3 florets
Fresh or frozen strawberries	½ cup	½ cup
Coffee *or* Tea	As desired	As desired

DINNER

Dry martini	None	1 martini
Steak squares on enriched toast points, with mushrooms	1 serving	1 serving
Broccoli with easy	2 stalks	2 stalks
Hollandaise sauce	1 tablespoon	1 tablespoon
Zucchini squash	½ cup	½ cup
Bibb lettuce *or* other salad greens	As desired	As desired
Lemon bread pudding	½ cup	½ cup
Milk	1 cup, non-fat	1 cup, whole

Friday

BREAKFAST	1,500 Calories	1,800 Calories
Apricot nectar	Scant ½ cup	Scant ½ cup
Egg poached in milk with	1 egg	1 egg
freshly ground pepper	2 tablespoons milk	2 tablespoons milk
English muffin	1 muffin	1 muffin
Butter	1 teaspoon	1 teaspoon
Coffee *or* Tea	As desired	As desired

LUNCHEON

	1,500 Calories	1,800 Calories
Oyster stew	1 serving	1 serving
skim milk	½ cup skim milk	½ cup skim milk
oysters	3-4 oysters	3-4 oysters
Crusty French bread	1 thick slice	1 thick slice
and herb butter	1 teaspoon	1 teaspoon
Green pepper strips	4 strips	4 strips
and tomato wedges	½ medium tomato	½ medium tomato
Apple pie	None	⅛ medium pie
Cheddar cheese cube	None	½-inch cube
Shiny red apple *or* fresh pear	1 medium	None
Camembert cheese	1 ounce	None
Coffee *or* Tea	As desired	As desired

DINNER

	1,500 Calories	1,800 Calories
Broiled fillet of salmon with	4 ounces before cooking	4 ounces before cooking
lemon-butter sauce	1 teaspoon butter	1 teaspoon butter
Fresh spinach	½ cup	½ cup
Cucumber, onion ring salad	As desired	As desired
Enriched Brown 'n Serve roll	1 roll	1 roll
Butter	1 teaspoon	1 teaspoon

Pound cake toast, topped with ice cream, with grated ginger	1 serving	1 serving
Pound cake	1 slice (3x2¾x⅝-inch)	1 slice (3x2¾x⅝-inch)
Ice cream	⅛ quart vanilla	⅛ quart vanilla
Grated ginger root	As desired	As desired
Milk	1 cup, non-fat	1 cup, whole

Saturday

BREAKFAST	*1,500 Calories*	*1,800 Calories*
Fresh grapefruit juice	Scant ½ cup	Scant ½ cup
One-egg omelet	1 serving	1 serving
Bacon	None	2 strips
Hot buttered toast	1 slice enriched bread	1 slice enriched bread
	1 teaspoon butter	1 teaspoon butter
Coffee *or* Tea	As desired	As desired

LUNCHEON		
Beef bouillon, chopped chives	As desired	As desired
Toasted turkey sandwich plate	1 serving	1 serving
enriched bread, toasted	2 slices	2 slices
butter	1 teaspoon	1 teaspoon
bacon bits	½ strip bacon	½ strip bacon
turkey	2 slices (3½x2⅝ x¼-inch)	2 slices (3½x2⅝ x¼-inch)
Cranberries	½ cup, ground	½ cup, ground
orange with	½ small, ground	½ small, ground
non-caloric sweetener on	As needed	As needed
escarole *or* salad greens	2 large leaves	2 large leaves
Caramel cupcake	1 medium	1 medium
Milk	1 cup, non-fat	1 cup, whole

DINNER

Scotch on the rocks	1½ ounces Scotch	1½ ounces Scotch
Baked pork chop marjoram	1 medium	2 medium
cheese-apple stuffing puff	½ cup	½ cup
Peas, Mandarin	1 serving	1 serving
peas	½ cup	½ cup
water chestnuts	2-3 water chestnuts	2-3 water chestnuts
Cabbage-grape salad	1 serving	1 serving
cabbage	½ cup, shredded	½ cup, shredded
Tokay grapes	8-10 grapes	8-10 grapes
Cloverleaf roll	None	1 enriched roll
butter	None	1 teaspoon
Fresh pineapple cubes	½ cup, unsweetened	½-cup, unsweetened
Coffee *or* Tea	As desired	As desired

PART VIII

FRESH, FROZEN AND CANNED FOODS USED INTERCHANGEABLY IN REDUCING DIETS

CHAPTER 25

Fresh Produce
Gives Diet Interest

WHETHER you use fresh, canned or frozen fruits and vegetables in your reducing diets is a matter of preference and availability only. However, for those who prefer fresh produce, today's markets offer an amazing array right through the year. Modern agricultural methods, pre-trimming and convenience packaging, rapid refrigerated transportation and improved methods of store display have turned the fresh produce department of your supermarket into a treasure trove of low-calorie and nutritionally rich eating pleasure.

Fresh salad greens are important for their fiber, consistency and pleasant taste. Large salads with calorie-free or low-calorie dressings, or with fresh lemon juice alone, give bulk to your reducing diets with only negligible amounts of calories. Eaten as a first course, they serve as mineral- and vitamin-rich appetite depressors for the remaining part of the meal.

Salad Greens Very Low in Calories

Among the salad greens with only a few calories are lettuce, watercress, dandelion, beet and turnip greens, the tender leaves of spinach, mustard greens, cabbage, chicory, escarole. Tomatoes, green peppers, radishes, celery, cucumbers, asparagus and raw mushrooms all make low-calorie and delicious additions to the salad bowl.

As between-meals low-calorie snacks, celery and radishes are excellent. Although they contain about 40 calories each, the following fresh fruits make low-calorie desserts and in-between-meals snacks: apples, bananas, blueberries and strawberries, oranges and grapefruit, peaches, pears, plums, cherries, fresh figs and tangerines. Keep a bowl of them handy to tempt the dieter away from richer desserts and more caloric snacks. Their color, shapes, consistency and fresh flavors will keep him happy though slender.

Seven-Day Diets Using Liberal Amounts of Fresh Fruits and Vegetables

(Daily Averages for Entire Week—1,300 Calories–2,000 Calories)

PREPARED BY:

Avanelle S. Day, M.S., Columbia University; member, American Dietetic Association.

Sunday

	Approximate Calories	Approximate Calories
BREAKFAST	*1,300*	*2,000*
Sliced fresh orange	1 medium	1 medium
Soft-cooked egg in shell	1 egg	2 eggs
Whole-wheat toast, thinly sliced	1 slice	2 slices
Butter *or* margarine	1 teaspoon	2 teaspoons
Black coffee		
LUNCH		
Grilled open-faced bacon and cheese sandwich	1	2
whole-wheat unbuttered bread	1 slice	2 slices
American cheese	1 slice	2 slices
crisp bacon	2 slices	4 slices
Relish tray		
celery		
carrot		

    cucumber

    tomato

Banana	1 medium	1 medium
Milk, non-fat, *or* buttermilk	8-ounce glass	8-ounce glass
Black coffee		

AFTERNOON OR BEDTIME SNACK

Grapes		1 small bunch

DINNER

Beef rib roast (each slice 3x2¼x¼-inch)	2 slices	3 slices
Riced potato	1 medium	1 medium
Butter *or* margarine	1 teaspoon	1 teaspoon
Sliced carrots braised with bouillon cube and water	½ cup	½ cup
Watercress, onion and radish salad with	as desired	as desired
French dressing	2 teaspoons	2 teaspoons
Rye bread		1 slice
cottage cheese		1 tablespoon
Baked apple, prepared with	1 medium	1 medium
sugar	2 teaspoons	2 teaspoons
Milk, non-fat, *or* buttermilk	8-ounce glass	8-ounce glass
Black coffee		

Monday

	Approximate Calories	*Approximate Calories*
BREAKFAST	*1,300*	*2,000*
Fresh orange juice	8-ounce glass	8-ounce glass
Cornflakes with	⅓ cup	1 cup
whole milk	¼ cup	½ cup
sugar	½ teaspoon	1 teaspoon
fresh grapes		⅔ cup
Rye toast	1 slice	1 slice
Butter *or* margarine	1 teaspoon	1 teaspoon
Black coffee		

LUNCH

Roast beef sandwich made with	1	1
roast beef, 3x2¼x¼-inch slices	2	2
whole-wheat bread, thinly sliced	2 slices	2 slices
butter *or* margarine	1 teaspoon	1 teaspoon
Grated carrot	1 medium	1 medium
Steamed banana custard, each serving ½ cup custard made with milk, non-fat, and ¼ large banana	6-ounce cup	6-ounce cup
Black coffee		

AFTERNOON OR BEDTIME SNACK

Fresh pear		1 medium

DINNER

Curried chicken broiled with butter	(¼ chicken, 1 teaspoon butter)	(½ chicken, 2 teaspoons butter)
Baked sliced potatoes, seasoned with	1 medium	1 medium
butter *or* margarine	1 teaspoon	1 teaspoon
Parsley zucchini squash and onion (cooked with bouillon cube)	½ cup	1 cup
Tomato, cucumber and spinach salad		
mayonnaise	1 teaspoon	1 teaspoon
Whole-wheat bread, thinly sliced		1 slice
cottage cheese		1 tablespoon
Fresh strawberries		½ cup
sugar		1 teaspoon

Plain cupcake, 2¾-inch di-
ameter   1
Milk, non-fat, *or* buttermilk   8-ounce glass   8-ounce glass
Black coffee

Tuesday

	Approximate Calories	Approximate Calories
BREAKFAST	**1,300**	**2,000**
Fresh grapefruit with	½ medium	½ medium
sugar	1 teaspoon	1 teaspoon
Coddled eggs	1 egg	2 eggs
Whole-wheat toast, thinly sliced	1 slice	2 slices
Butter *or* margarine	1 teaspoon	2 teaspoons
Black coffee		

LUNCH

Corned beef hash	½ cup	1 cup
Parsley diced carrots	½ cup	½ cup
Tossed green salad with French dressing	2 teaspoons	2 teaspoons
Whole-wheat bread, thinly sliced	1 slice	1 slice
cottage cheese	1 tablespoon	1 tablespoon
Grapes		1 small bunch
Milk, non-fat, *or* buttermilk	8-ounce glass	8-ounce glass

AFTERNOON OR BEDTIME SNACK

Fresh orange		1 medium

DINNER

Shoulder of veal roast without bone	3 ounces	3 ounces
Baked potato with	1 medium	1 medium
sour cream and chives	2 teaspoons	2 teaspoons

Herbed steamed fresh kale with lemon juice	½ cup	1 cup
Cole slaw	½ cup	½ cup
Whole-wheat bread, thinly sliced	1 slice	2 slices
cottage cheese	1 tablespoon	2 tablespoons
Fresh fruit cup		½ cup
Plain cookie, 3x½-inch		2 cookies
Milk, non-fat, *or* buttermilk	8-ounce glass	8-ounce glass
Black coffee		

Wednesday

	Approximate Calories	Approximate Calories
BREAKFAST	*1,300*	*2,000*
Fresh cantaloupe	½ medium	½ medium
40% bran flakes with	¾ cup	1 cup
whole milk	¼ cup	⅓ cup
sugar	½ teaspoon	1 teaspoon
Whole-wheat toast, thinly sliced	1 slice	2 slices
Butter *or* margarine	1 teaspoon	2 teaspoons
Milk, whole		6-ounce glass
Black coffee		

LUNCH		
Hamburger on bun	1 large	1 large
Mixed salad greens with French dressing	2 teaspoons	2 teaspoons
Fresh orange sections	½ cup	½ cup
Milk, non-fat, *or* buttermilk	8-ounce glass	8-ounce glass
Black coffee		

AFTERNOON OR BEDTIME SNACK		
Fresh apple		1 medium
Sugar cookie		1

DINNER

Calves' liver, 3x2¼x⅜-inch slices (broiled with butter or margarine)	2 slices 1 teaspoon	2 slices 1 teaspoon
Mashed potatoes with milk, non-fat	½ cup	1 cup
Steamed broccoli with fresh lemon juice	½ cup	½ cup
Tossed lettuce salad with French dressing	2 teaspoons	2 teaspoons
Whole-wheat bread, thinly sliced		2 slices
cottage cheese		2 tablespoons
Fresh grapefruit with	½ medium	½ medium
sugar or	1 teaspoon	
lemon sherbet		1 small scoop
Milk, non-fat, or buttermilk	8-ounce glass	8-ounce glass
Black coffee		

Thursday

	Approximate Calories	Approximate Calories
BREAKFAST	*1,300*	*2,000*
Fresh grapefruit with	½ medium	½ medium
sugar	1 teaspoon	1 teaspoon
Poached egg on toast (1 egg, 1 slice whole-wheat toast)	1 serving	1 serving
Crisp bacon	1 slice	2 slices
Raisin toast		1 slice
Butter or margarine		1 teaspoon
Black coffee		

LUNCH

Cream of celery soup	¾ cup	1 cup
Saltines	2	2
Fresh apple, grape and cottage cheese salad		

apple	¼ medium	¼ medium
grapes	¼ cup	¼ cup
cottage cheese	⅓ cup	⅓ cup
lettuce		
mayonnaise	1 teaspoon	1 teaspoon
Boston brown bread	1 slice, 3x½-inch	2 slices, 3x½-inch
Butter *or* margarine	1 teaspoon	2 teaspoons
Black coffee		

AFTERNOON OR BEDTIME SNACK

Banana		1 medium
Milk, non-fat, *or* buttermilk	8-ounce glass	8-ounce glass

DINNER

Rib lamb chops	2	2
Dill potatoes with	1 medium	1 medium
butter *or* margarine	1 teaspoon	1 teaspoon
Steamed fresh spinach with lemon juice	½ cup	½ cup
Fresh tomatoes	3 slices	3 slices
Whole-wheat bread, thinly sliced	1 slice	2 slices
cottage cheese	1 tablespoon	2 tablespoons
Jellied fresh orange juice and banana cup (½ cup fresh orange juice, ¼ medium banana, 1½ teaspoons sugar and unflavored gelatin)	1 serving	1 serving
Milk, non-fat, *or* buttermilk	8-ounce glass	8-ounce glass
Black coffee		

Friday

	Approximate Calories	Approximate Calories
BREAKFAST	*1,300*	*2,000*
Fresh orange and apple cup	1 serving	1 serving
fresh orange sections	½ cup	½ cup

diced fresh apples	⅓ cup	⅓ cup
Oatmeal with	½ cup	1 cup
whole milk	¼ cup	⅓ cup
sugar	1 teaspoon	1½ teaspoons
Whole-wheat toast, thinly sliced	1 slice	2 slices
Butter *or* margarine	1 teaspoon	2 teaspoons
Black coffee		

LUNCH

Fresh pear and carrot salad	1 serving	1 serving
pear	1 medium	1 medium
grated carrot	½ cup	½ cup
lettuce leaves	2 leaves	2 leaves
mayonnaise	1 teaspoon	1 teaspoon
Corned beef	3 ounces	3 ounces
Rye toast	1 slice	1 slice
cottage cheese	1 tablespoon	1 tablespoon
Milk, non-fat, *or* buttermilk	8-ounce glass	8-ounce glass
Black coffee		

AFTERNOON OR BEDTIME SNACK

Grapes		1 small bunch
Milk, non-fat, *or* buttermilk	8-ounce glass	8-ounce glass

DINNER

Broiled shrimp with	½ cup	½ cup
butter	1 teaspoon	1 teaspoon
fresh lemon juice	1 teaspoon	1 teaspoon
Parsley potato	1 medium	1 medium
sour cream	2 teaspoons	2 teaspoons
Green peas	⅓ cup	½ cup
Curried broiled tomato with	½ medium	½ medium
butter *or* margarine	1 teaspoon	1 teaspoon
Whole-wheat bread, thinly sliced	1 slice	2 slices
cottage cheese	1 tablespoon	2 tablespoons
Gingerbread, 2½x2½x2-inch	1 square	1 square

square with		
banana	⅛ medium	⅛ medium
whipped cream		2 teaspoons
Milk, non-fat, *or* buttermilk	8-ounce glass	8-ounce glass
Black coffee		

Saturday

	Approximate Calories	*Approximate Calories*
BREAKFAST	1,300	2,000
Sliced fresh orange	1 medium	1 medium
Poached egg on toast (1 egg, 1 slice whole-wheat toast)	1 serving	2 servings
Crisp bacon		2 slices
Black coffee		
LUNCH		
Banana salad	1 serving	1 serving
banana	1 medium	1 medium
lettuce	2 leaves	2 leaves
mayonnaise	1 teaspoon	1 teaspoon
Cottage cheese	½ cup	½ cup
Crisp celery	as desired	as desired
Rye wafer, double squares	1 double square	2 double squares
Sponge cake, 2-inch sector of 8-inch cake	1 serving	1 serving
Milk, non-fat, *or* buttermilk	8-ounce glass	8-ounce glass
Black coffee		
AFTERNOON OR BEDTIME SNACK		
Fresh apple		1 medium
Milk, non-fat, *or* buttermilk	8-ounce glass	8-ounce glass
DINNER		
Boiled tongue	4 ounces	4 ounces
Baked potato with	1 medium	1 medium
sour cream	1 tablespoon	1 tablespoon

Steamed cabbage wedge with fresh lemon juice and caraway seeds	1 serving	1 serving
Watercress and tomato salad	1 serving	1 serving
tomato	3 slices	3 slices
French dressing	2 teaspoons	2 teaspoons
Rye bread, thinly sliced	1 slice	2 slices
cottage cheese	1 tablespoon	2 tablespoons
Diced fresh pineapple	½ cup	½ cup
sugar	1 teaspoon	1 teaspoon
fresh lemon juice	1 teaspoon	1 teaspoon
Wafers, 2½-inch	1 wafer	2 wafers
Milk, non-fat, or buttermilk	8-ounce glass	8-ounce glass
Black coffee		

CHAPTER 26

Canned Foods
Simplify
Diet Menus

MODERN technology has improved canned foods to so high a degree that they are now nutritionally the equal of fresh foods. Therefore, the dieter can use them liberally in his menus.

The small-sized cans, containing one or two servings, are excellent choices for the dieter who lives alone. They prevent waste and also make variety more practical than do the large cans.

Many fruits and vegetables are canned without sugar, or with artificial sweeteners. These are the best choice for very low-calorie diets.

Seven-Day 1,500-Calorie and 2,200-Calorie Diets with Liberal Use of Canned Foods

PREPARED BY:

Katherine R. Smith, B.S., in Foods and Nutrition, University of Minnesota; member, American Dietetic Association.

Gloria Hansen, B.S., in Foods and Nutrition, Iowa State College; member, American Home Economics Association.

Sunday

1,500 CALORIES	2,200 CALORIES
BREAKFAST	
Sliced orange, medium-sized	
Scrambled egg, 1	2 eggs

Canadian bacon, 1 slice   2 slices
Popover, 1   2 popovers
Apple jelly, 1 tablespoon   and 1 pat butter
Milk, non-fat, 1 cup   whole milk, 1 cup
Coffee, black

LUNCHEON OR SUPPER

Crabmeat salad
  canned crabmeat, ½ cup
  hard-cooked egg, ½
  green onions, 3
  radishes, 3
  lettuce, 3 leaves
  Russian salad dressing, 1 tablespoon
Cracked-wheat bread, ½ slice   1 slice
Butter, ½ pat   1 pat
Milk, non-fat, 1 cup   whole milk, 1 cup

DINNER

Baked canned ham, 4 ounces
Buttered green beans and
  mushrooms, ¾ cup
Mashed squash, ½ cup
Relishes:
  celery, 2 3-inch stalks
  carrot strips, ½ carrot
  ripe olives, 2 large
Roll, 1 medium   2 rolls
Butter, ½ pat   1 pat
Sherbet-Peach Sundae:
  1 large canned peach half
  ¼ cup raspberry sherbet   2 small macaroons
Coffee, black

PICK-UP SNACK, AFTERNOON OR EVENING

1 6-ounce glass tomato juice

Monday

1,500 CALORIES	2,200 CALORIES

BREAKFAST

Orange-grapefruit juice, canned, 4 ounces
Poached egg, 1   2 eggs
Toast, white bread, 1 slice   2 slices
Butter, ½ pat   1 pat
Milk, non-fat, 1 cup   whole milk, 1 cup
Coffee, black

LUNCHEON

Cream of tomato soup, ¾ cup
Open chicken sandwich   add 1 pat butter
   whole-wheat bread, 1 slice
   canned, boned chicken, 2 ounces
   low-calorie salad dressing, 1 tablespoon
Baked apple, 1 large, 1 tablespoon sugar
Coffee, black, *or* Tea

DINNER

New England boiled dinner
   Corned beef, 1 slice 7x2x¼-inch   2 slices corned beef
   canned potatoes, 3-4 small
   cabbage, 1 wedge
   carrot, 1 medium-sized
Celery sticks, 3, 5 inches long
Corn stick   2 corn sticks
Butter, ½ pat   1 pat
Apricots, canned, 4 medium halves
Sugar cookie, 1   2 sugar cookies
Coffee, black

PICK-UP SNACK, AFTERNOON OR EVENING

1 8-ounce glass non-fat milk *or* buttermilk

Tuesday

1,500 CALORIES	2,200 CALORIES

BREAKFAST

Grapefruit sections, canned, ½ cup
Egg, soft-cooked, 1
Bacon, crisp, 1 slice — 2 slices
Toast, whole-wheat bread, 1 slice — 2 slices
Butter, ½ pat — 1 pat
Milk, non-fat, *or* buttermilk, 1 cup — whole milk, 1 cup
Coffee, black

LUNCHEON

Broiled hamburger, 4 ounces
Toasted hamburger roll — add 1 pat butter
Relish plate
  dill pickle, 1 large
  celery hearts, 3 small
  radish roses, 2 small
  carrot sticks, 1 small carrot
Coconut bar cookies, 3 — 4 cookies
Milk, non-fat, *or* buttermilk, 1 cup — whole milk, 1 cup

DINNER

Tomato juice, 4 ounces
Roast leg of lamb, 3 ounces
Baked potato, 1 medium — 1 large
Asparagus, canned, 6 medium spears
Tossed green salad
  mixed greens, 1½ cups
  garlic French dressing, 1 tablespoon

1 slice French bread
Butter, 1 pat — 2 pats butter
Strawberries, 1 cup, 2 tablespoons sugar — strawberry shortcake
Whipped cream, scant tablespoon
Coffee, black

PICK-UP SNACK, AFTERNOON OR EVENING

1 cup canned beef broth, hot or over ice

Wednesday

1,500 CALORIES

2,200 CALORIES

BREAKFAST

Cantaloupe, ½ melon
Bran flakes, ¾ cup
Toast, raisin bread, 1 slice   2 slices
Butter, ½ pat   1 pat
Marmalade, 1 teaspoon

     2 slices crisp bacon
Milk, non-fat, 1 cup   whole milk, 1 cup
Coffee, black

LUNCHEON

Frankfurter, 1   2 frankfurters
Mashed potatoes, ½ cup
Sauerkraut, canned, ½ cup
Carrot sticks, 1 small carrot
Whole-wheat bread, 1 slice
Pears, canned, 2 halves

     pound cake, 1 average slice
Tea with lemon

DINNER

Broiled sirloin steak, 4 ounces   6-ounce serving
Broccoli, ⅔ cup or 1 large stalk
Butter browned sweet potatoes, ½ cup
Salad
     lettuce, ⅙ head
     tomato, medium size, 3 slices
     low-calorie French dressing, 2 tablespoons
French bread, 1 slice   with 1 pat butter
Baked custard, ½ cup
Coffee, black

PICK-UP SNACK, AFTERNOON OR EVENING

2 celery stalks stuffed with
     seasoned cottage cheese

Thursday

1,500 CALORIES	2,200 CALORIES

BREAKFAST

Orange juice, canned, 6 ounces	
Scrambled egg, 1	2 eggs
Corn muffin	2 muffins
Butter, ½ pat	1 pat
Milk, non-fat, 1 cup	
Coffee, black	

LUNCHEON

Consommé, 1 cup	
Salmon Salad Plate	
canned salmon, ½ cup	
cottage cheese, ½ cup	
tomato, 1 medium-sized	
Crisp rye wafer, 1 square	double square
	1 pat butter
Tea, plain	whole milk, 1 cup

DINNER

Broiled chicken, ¼ chicken	½ chicken
Buttered green beans, canned, ½ cup	
Buttered whole kernel corn, canned, ½ cup	
Cole slaw, ⅔ cup	
Parkerhouse roll, 1	
Butter, ½ pat	1 pat butter
Angel food cake, 1 average size serving	
Coffee, black	

PICK-UP SNACK, AFTERNOON OR EVENING

   1 8-ounce glass non-fat milk *or* buttermilk

Friday

1,500 CALORIES   **2,200 CALORIES**

BREAKFAST

Grapefruit sections, canned, ½ cup
Oatmeal, ½ cup, 1 teaspoon sugar
Toast, whole-wheat bread, 1 slice   2 slices
Butter, ½ pat   1 pat
Milk, non-fat, 1 cup   whole milk, 1 cup
Coffee, black

LUNCHEON

Herb omelet, 2 eggs
Tomatoes, cold or hot, canned, ½ cup
Toasted roll, ½   whole roll
                                           1 pat butter
Milk, non-fat, 1 cup   hot chocolate
                                           with 2 fig bars

Pineapple gelatin mold
  lemon gelatin, 3 ounces
  crushed pineapple, 2 ounces

DINNER

Broiled flounder or Sole, 3x3x⅜-inch
Butter browned potatoes, canned, 3-4 small
Beets vinegarette, canned, ½ cup
Asparagus, canned, 6 medium spears
Mixed salad:
  endive *or* chicory, 10 leaves
  lettuce, 2 large leaves
  cauliflowerets, raw, ¼ cup
  low-calorie French dressing, 2 tablespoons
                                           cloverleaf roll
                                           1 pat butter
Apple Brown Betty, scant ½ cup
Whipped cream, scant tablespoon   heaping tablespoon
Coffee, black

PICK-UP SNACK, AFTERNOON OR EVENING

　　1 4-ounce glass apricot nectar, 2 saltine crackers

Saturday

1,500 CALORIES

2,200 CALORIES

BREAKFAST

　　Tomato juice, 6 ounces
　　Corn flakes, ¾ cup
　　Banana, ½ small
　　Milk, non-fat, 1 cup

　　　　　　　　　　　　　　　　　whole milk, 1 cup
　　　　　　　　　　　　　　　　　1 slice white toast
　　　　　　　　　　　　　　　　　1 pat butter
　　　　　　　　　　　　　　　　　poached egg, 1

　　Coffee, black

LUNCHEON

　　　　　　　　　　　　　　　　　vegetable-beef soup
　　　　　　　　　　　　　　　　　saltine crackers, 3

　　Tuna sandwich
　　　　white toast, 2 slices
　　　　lettuce, 2 leaves
　　　　tuna, 2 ounces, mixed with celery and onion
　　　　salad dressing, 1 tablespoon
　　Sweet pickles, 2 small
　　Applesauce, canned, sweetened, ½ cup
　　Tea with lemon

　　　　　　　　　　　　　　　　　whole milk, 1 cup

DINNER

　　Broiled loin lamb chop, 4-ounce　　mixed grill:
　　　　　　　　　　　　　　　　　loin lamp chop, 4 ounce
　　　　　　　　　　　　　　　　　calves' liver, 2 ounces

　　Baked potato, medium size
　　Peas paprika, canned, ½ cup
　　Spartan salad
　　　　grapefruit sections, 3
　　　　spinach, 1 cup

low-calorie salad dressing, 1 table-
    spoon
Parkerhouse roll, 1
Butter, ½ pat   Butter, 1 pat
Lemon sponge cake, 1 average size
    serving
Coffee, black

PICK-UP SNACK, AFTERNOON OR EVENING

1 4-ounce glass vegetable juice
   cocktail
1 saltine cracker, ½ ounce cheddar   2 saltines, ½ ounce cheese
   cheese

CHAPTER 27

Frozen Foods
Convenient in Diets

FROZEN FOODS can be used in place of fresh or canned whenever the dieter desires. If they make meal preparation easier, and if their variety adds interest, then they are a boon to the dieter in encouraging him to stay within his calorie budget and be happy at the same time.

Seven-Day 1,500-Calorie Diet with Liberal Use of Frozen Foods

PREPARED BY:

Eva D. Wilson, Ph.D., in Nutrition and Physiology, University of Chicago; professor of Nutrition, Pennsylvania State University; member, American Dietetic Association.

Sunday

BREAKFAST

Frozen orange juice	½ cup
Butter *or* Margarine	1 pat (½ tablespoon)
Toast	1 slice
Frozen breaded, cooked fish sticks	2
Coffee, black	

DINNER

Hot or cold bouillon	1 cup
Roast leg of lamb, without bone	3 ounces
Frozen mashed potatoes	½ cup

Frozen peas cooked with mint extract	½ cup
Tomato and lettuce salad	
Medium tomato	½
Lettuce leaves	4
French dressing	1 tablespoon
Sherbet	
with frozen sweetened peaches	½ cup
Coffee, black	¼ cup

SUPPER

Frozen cooked broccoli spears in	1 cup, or 3 large spears
cheese sauce—white sauce	¼ cup
cheese	½-inch cube
Dry toast, 1 slice	
Fruit-flavored gelatin whipped	⅓ cup
with frozen sweetened whole strawberries	¼ cup
Hot tea, no sugar	
Milk, non-fat	1 cup
Total Calories	1,522
With frozen cherry pie, 1 piece	1,862

Monday

BREAKFAST

Grapefruit	½ medium
Bacon, drained after cooking	2 slices
Frozen French toast	1 slice
Jelly	1 tablespoon
Egg, poached	1
Coffee, black	

LUNCH

Open-faced sandwich of	
toasted bread	1 slice
lunch meat	2 ounces

cheese, melted	1 ounce
Apple, medium	1
Cookie	1
Milk, non-fat	1 cup

DINNER

Frozen main course of meat loaf	2½ ounces
with tomato sauce	½ cup
with frozen green beans	½ cup
Butter with beans	½ pat
Frozen French fried potatoes	½ cup
Cucumber and lettuce salad	
French dressing	1 tablespoon
Frozen raspberries and	½ cup
banana	½
Coffee, black	
Milk, non-fat	1 cup
Total Calories, approximately	1,521
With frozen frosted cake, 1 piece	1,826

Tuesday

BREAKFAST

Frozen strawberries, whole, sweetened	½ cup
Sausage links, cooked and drained	2
Frozen waffles, toasted	2 small
Butter *or* Margarine	1 teaspoon
Syrup	1 tablespoon
Coffee, black	

LUNCH

Frozen vegetable with beef soup	1 cup
Cottage cheese on lettuce	½ cup
Bran muffin	1
Butter *or* Margarine	1 teaspoon
Applesauce, spiced	½ cup
Tea	
Milk, non-fat	1 cup

DINNER

Frozen grapefruit juice	½ cup
Frozen roast turkey	2 slices
Frozen mashed potatoes	½ cup
Frozen cauliflower	
Salad greens, lemon juice dressing	
Custard	½ cup
Coffee, black	

Total Calories   1,592

With substitution of frozen turkey with mashed potatoes and dressing for sliced turkey and mashed potatoes, and one serving of ice cream for custard, and addition of 2 saltines, the total calories will be 1,782.

Wednesday

Corn flakes *or* other prepared cereal	1 cup
with frozen unsweetened blueberries	½ cup
Sugar	1 teaspoon
Milk, whole	½ cup
Soft-cooked egg	1
Toast	1 slice
Butter *or* Margarine	1 teaspoon
Coffee, black	

LUNCH

Tomato soup	1 cup
Frozen grilled sandwich steaks, no fat added	3 ounces
Toast	1 slice
Banana	1 medium
Tea	
Milk, non-fat	1 cup

DINNER

| Casserole of frozen corn | ½ cup |
| with frozen oysters | ¼ cup |

cream sauce, thin	½ cup
Frozen French fried potatoes	½ cup
Mixed green salad	
Frozen pineapple chunks	½ cup
Sponge cake	1-inch section
Coffee, black	

| Total Calories | 1,536 |

With addition of 1 hard roll, ½ teaspoon butter or margarine, 2 tablespoons light cream with coffee and 2 saltine crackers, the total calories will be 1,737.

Thursday

BREAKFAST

Frozen grape juice	½ cup
Cereal, cooked	½ cup
Milk, whole	¼ cup
Sugar	1 teaspoon
Muffin, plain	1
Butter *or* Margarine	1 teaspoon
Coffee, black	

LUNCH

Hot tomato juice	½ cup
Frozen haddock, broiled	
Roll	1
Butter *or* Margarine	½ pat
Lettuce	¼ head
Baked frozen, sweetened rhubarb	½ cup
Tea	
Milk, non-fat	1 cup

DINNER

Beef pot roast frozen dinner	
beef, without bone	3 ounces
gravy	¼ cup
potato, browned	1 medium

Frozen succotash	½ cup
Butter	1 teaspoon
Frozen peas	½ cup
Carrot sticks	
Cantaloupe	½
Coffee, black	
Milk, non-fat	1 cup
Total Calories	1,577

With 1 roll, ½ teaspoon butter and 1 serving of ice cream, the total calories will be 1,846.

Friday

BREAKFAST

Frozen grapefruit and orange juice	½ cup
Frozen pancake	1
Butter *or* Margarine	1 teaspoon
Syrup	1 tablespoon
Canadian bacon, 2¼x3/16-inch	2 slices
Coffee, black	

LUNCH

Frozen macaroni and cheese casserole	⅔ cup
Frozen peach slices on lettuce	½ cup
Roll	1
Butter *or* Margarine	1 teaspoon
Tea	
Milk, non-fat	1 cup

DINNER

Broiled frozen buttered beef patties *or* Halibut cooked in butter-lemon sauce	
Frozen asparagus	½ cup
Tomato slices	
Frozen unsweetened blueberries with soft custard	1 cup
Coffee, black	
Milk, non-fat	

Total Calories   1,539

With 1 large glass sweetened lemonade; a second frozen pancake and 1 cookie, the total calories will be 1,808.

Saturday

BREAKFAST

Frozen peach slices	½ cup
Cereal, dry	1 cup
Milk, whole	¼ cup
Egg, poached	1
Toast	½ slice
Butter or Margarine	1 teaspoon
Coffee	

LUNCH

Frankfurter	1
Bun	1
Apple and celery salad	
mayonnaise	1 tablespoon
Tea	
Milk, non-fat	1 cup

DINNER

Frozen cream of shrimp soup	½ cup
Green salad with frozen mixed vegetables and cheese	
Mayonnaise	1 tablespoon
Corn muffin	
Butter *or* Margarine	½ teaspoon
Fruit-flavored gelatin	
Milk, non-fat	1 cup

Total Calories   1,550

With ½ slice toast, 1 tablespoon catsup, 1 slice frozen pound cake and ½ cup frozen sweetened raspberries, the total calories will be 1,720.

BIBLIOGRAPHY

ADVANCES IN NUTRITION: Charles Glen King. *Jour. Amer. Dietetic Assoc.*, Vol. 35, No. 2, 1959.

ATHEROSCLEROSIS AND THE FAT CONTENT OF THE DIET: Irvine H. Page, Fredrick J. Stare, A. C. Corcoran, Herbert Pollack and Charles F. Wilkinson. *Jour. Amer. Medical Assoc.*, Vol. 164, August 31, 1957.

BEEF CAN BE EVERYBODY'S MEAT: Fredrick J. Stare. *McCall's*, March, 1957.

BETTER MEALS MAKE BETTER FAMILIES: 12 articles, Gaynor Maddox. Newspaper Enterprise Association, Inc., September, 1959.

BIOLOGY OF STARVATION: Ancel Keys, et al. University of Minnesota Press, 1950.

CHANGING ATTITUDES TOWARD OVERWEIGHT AND REDUCING: Winifred M. Ayers. *Jour. Amer. Dietetic Assoc.*, Vol. 34, No. 1, 1958.

COMPOSITION OF FOODS: U.S. Dept. of Agriculture. Agriculture Handbook No. 8.

DAILY FOOD GUIDE: U.S. Dept. of Agriculture. Leaflet No. 424.

DIABETES—OVERWEIGHT: U.S. PROBLEMS: James M. Hundley, M.D. *Jour. Amer. Dietetic Assoc.*, Vol. 32, No. 5, 1956.

DIET, DRUGS AND DEVICES: *Consumer Reports*, February, 1958.

DIET FATS AND ADULT HEALTH: Ancel Keys, Ph.D., and Paul Dudley White, M.D. *Nutrition News*, Vol. 20, No. 1, 1956.

DIETARY FATS AND ATHEROSCLEROSIS: T. B. Van Itallie. *Nutrition Reviews*, 15:1-6, 1957 (January).

EAT WELL AND STAY WELL: Ancel and Margaret Keys. Doubleday, 1959.

EFFECT OF WEIGHT LOSS ON BLOOD PRESSURE: J. V. Salzano, Ruth Gunning, T. N. Mastopaulo, W. W. Tuttle. *Jour. Amer. Dietetic Assoc.*, Vol. 34, No. 12, 1958.

EMOTIONAL FACTORS IN OBESITY AND WEIGHT REDUCTION: C. D. Darling, M.D., and John Summerskill, Ph.D. *Jour. Amer. Dietetic Assoc.*, Vol. 29, No. 12, 1953.

ENERGY VALUE OF FOODS: U.S. Dept. of Agriculture. Agriculture Handbook No. 74.

FATHER'S INFLUENCE ON YOUNG CHILDREN'S FOOD PREFERENCE: Marian S. Bryan and Miriam E. Lowenberg, Ph.D. *Jour. Amer. Dietetic Assoc.*, Vol. 34, No. 1, 1958.

FATS IN NUTRITION AND HEALTH: Charles Glen King. *Jour. Amer. Oil Chemists Society,* Vol. XXXIV, No. 11, 1957.

FATS MAKE GOOD FOODS—WHERE AND WHY ARE THE MARGINS?: Charles Glen King. *Food Technology,* Vol. XIII, No. 1, 1959.

FOOD: Yearbook of Agriculture, 1959. U.S. Dept. of Agriculture.

FOOD BECOMES YOU: Ruth M. Leverton. University of Nebraska Press, 1952.

FOOD FACTS TALK BACK (booklet): American Dietetic Association. 1957.

FOOD INTAKES OF OBESE AND NON-OBESE WOMEN: Rachel Beaudoin, D.Sc., and J. Mayer, Ph.D., D.Sc. *Jour. Amer. Dietetic Assoc.,* Vol. 29, No. 1, 1953.

FOOD VALUES OF PORTIONS COMMONLY USED: Anna de Planter Bowes and Charles F. Church. Published by Mrs. Anna de Planter Bowes, Philadelphia. 8th edition, 1956.

FOODS AND HEALTH ARE CLOSE TO YOUR HEART: Charles Glen King. *AMA Archives of Industrial Health,* Vol. 17, May, 1958.

GROUP DISCUSSION IN CHANGING FOOD HABITS: Edward C. Norman, M.D. *Jour. Amer. Dietetic Assoc.,* Vol. 34, No. 11, 1958.

HANDBOOK OF DIET THERAPY: Dorothea F. Turner. University of Chicago Press. 2nd revision, 1959.

HOW HEALTHFUL IS EXERCISE?: *Consumer Reports,* October, 1959.

HOW TO CONTROL YOUR WEIGHT: Metropolitan Life Insurance Co. 1958.

HOW TO LOSE WEIGHT: Donald Cooley. Random House, 1956.

HOW TO REDUCE SURELY AND SAFELY: Herbert Pollack, M.D. McGraw-Hill, 1955.

IMPORTANCE OF OVERWEIGHT: Hilda Bruck, M.D. Norton, 1957.

LONG-TERM EFFECT OF WEIGHT-REDUCING PROGRAMS: Mary McCann and Martha F. Trulson. *Jour. Amer. Dietetic Assoc.,* Vol. 31, No. 11, 1108-1110; 1955.

METABOLIC DEMANDS AS A FACTOR IN WEIGHT CONTROL: Herbert Pollack, M.D., C. Frank Consolagio and Gerhard J. Isaac. *Jour. Amer. Medical Assoc.,* Vol. 167, May 10, 1958.

MODIFYING THE FATTY ACID CONTENT OF THE DIET: Patricia A. Stefanik and Martha F. Trulson. *Jour. Amer. Dietetic Assoc.,* Vol. 34, No. 6, 1958.

NIGHT-EATING SYNDROME: Albert J. Stunkard, M.D., William J. Grace, M.D., and Harold G. Wolff, M.D. *Amer. Jour. of Medicine,* Vol. XIX, No. 1, 1955.

NO-FAD DIET: 6 articles, Gaynor Maddox. Newspaper Enterprise Association, January, 1958.

NO-NONSENSE DIET: 6 articles, Gaynor Maddox. Newspaper Enterprise Association, January, 1959.

NON-CALORIC SWEETENERS AND WEIGHT REDUCTION: Mary B. McCann, Martha F. Trulson and Sarah C. Stulb. *Jour. Amer. Dietetic Assoc.*, Vol. 32, No. 4, 1956.

NUTRITIONAL PROBLEMS OF ADVANCING AGE: Fredrick J. Stare. *Bulletin, N. Y. Academy of Medicine*, Vol. 32, No. 4, 1956.

NUTRITIVE VALUE OF COOKED MEAT: Ruth M. Leverton and George V. Odell. Oklahoma State University. Miscellaneous Publication MP-49, March, 1958.

PROBLEM OF THE OBESE PATIENT: Charlotte M. Young. *Jour. Amer. Dietetic Assoc.*, Vol. 31, No. 11, 1955.

PROCEEDINGS OF BORDEN CENTENNIAL SYMPOSIUM ON NUTRITION: Borden Company Foundation. 1958.

PSYCHOLOGIC FACTORS IN WEIGHT CONTROL: Charlotte M. Young, Ph.D., Kathleen Berresford, M.S., and Norman S. Moore, M.D. *Amer. Jour. of Clinical Nutrition*, Vol. 5, No. 2, 1957.

PSYCHOLOGICAL IMPACT OF DIET RESTRICTION: Justin Simon, M.D. American Dietetic Association, August, 1959.

PSYCHOLOGY OF WEIGHT REDUCTION: Walter W. Hamburger, M.D. *Jour. Amer. Dietetic Assoc.*, Vol. 34, No. 1, 1958.

RECOMMENDED DIETARY ALLOWANCES, revised 1958: National Research Council. Publication 589.

REDUCE AND STAY REDUCED: Norman Jolliffe, M.D. Simon and Schuster, 1957.

RELATIVE IMPORTANCE OF INACTIVITY AND OVEREATING IN THE ENERGY BALANCE OF OBESE HIGH SCHOOL GIRLS: Mary Louise Johnson, D.Sc., Bertha S. Burke, M.A., and J. Mayer, Ph.D., D.Sc. *Amer. Jour. of Clinical Nutrition*, Vol. 4, No. 1, 1955.

ROUND NUMBER BARRIER IN WEIGHT REDUCTION: Leonid Kotkin, M.D. *N. Y. State Jour. of Medicine*, Vol. 55, No. 1, 1955.

SIMPLE OBESITY: George H. Berryman. *Jour. Amer. Dietetic Assoc.*, Vol. 31, No. 4, 1955.

STAY SLIM FOR LIFE: Ida Jean Kain and Mildred B. Gibson. Doubleday, 1958.

STRESS OF LIFE: Hans Selye, M.D. McGraw-Hill, 1956.

WEIGHT CONTROL: Weight Control Colloquium. Iowa State College Press, 1955.

WEIGHT CONTROL, A COMMUNITY PROGRAM: June Boss Yule, Ethel L. Marth and Charlotte M. Young, Ph.D. *Jour. Amer. Dietetic Assoc.*, Vol. 33, No. 1, 1957.

WEIGHT CONTROL THROUGH PREVENTION OF OBESITY: W. H. Sebrell, Jr., M.D. *Jour. Amer. Dietetic Assoc.*, Vol. 34, No. 9, 1958.

WHAT WE KNOW ABOUT DIET AND HEART DISEASE: American Heart Association. 1958.

WHY YOU GET FAT: 6 articles, Gaynor Maddox. Newspaper Enterprise Association, February, 1957.

WORLD SEARCH FOR GOOD QUALITY PROTEINS: Charles Glen King. *Food Technology,* Vol. XI, No. 2, 1957.

GAYNOR MADDOX, the world's most widely read writer on food and nutrition, believes that being fat is as crippling as fearing to live zestfully. His annual six-part series for the Newspaper Enterprise Association, on scientific weight control with human overtones, has established him as the most persuasive liaison between research laboratories and the family bathroom scales. He is in daily contact with physicians, biochemists and dietitians, food industrialists and agriculturists.

Food and Markets Editor of NEA, Mr. Maddox is considered by scientists one of the most accurate and talented writers on nutrition. His book, EAT WELL FOR LESS MONEY, articles in national magazines, and lectures have increased his prestige

Mr. Maddox has long been insatiably curious about the effects of food on health, emotions and politics. His curiosity has taken him not only to the world's great restaurants and clubs, but to forecastles, cabooses and working men's homes. He has eaten in waterfront dives in Yokohama and Nagasaki, shared near-starvation meals in coolie huts and on sampans in China, with untouchables in India and peons on Latin American banana plantations.

Born in California, Gaynor Maddox was educated at the University of California and at Harvard. Life-loving, internationally known, he lives in New York City with his wife and teen-age son, and is now at work on his third book about food and life.